Dill *icio*
Veg

A variety of sweet & savoury dishes for every occasion

Easy enough even for the beginner

Erasmia Kyriakou

Acknowledgements

Thank you to everyone who has supported me on this journey of mine.

To my grandmother and mother for passing down their knowledge and passion for cooking and baking, they have both been a huge inspiration in my life and taught me everything I know. Also, thanks to my aunts and sisters for sharing their recipes, for their kind advice and support. Thank you all so much, I am truly grateful to you all and love you all dearly xx.

To all the lovely people I have met in my cafe, thank you all for your kind words, constant support and for being as excited about my book as I am! The wonderful girls at work for giving me some time off to finish the book, thank you x.

Ness, my darling thanks for all your help and advice on photography and lighting! Your tips helped me more than you know. Thanks to you I got the photos done. I appreciate you for being the wonderful person you are and for always making me laugh x.

Last but not least, my dearest Claire, for helping me with my introduction and proofreading my book and of course for tasting most of the recipes and giving me good honest feedback on each one. Thank you for being there with me and motivating me to keep going. Your advice and belief in me has helped me a great deal in finishing the book xxx.

Thank you all very much! I could never have done it without all the amazing people in my life, you were there to give me help and support. I feel very lucky and remain thankful that this day has finally come when my dream became a reality.

I hope you all enjoy this book as much as I enjoyed creating it xxx

Follow my books at Dill_iciously_Vegan.

www.instagram.com/dill_iciously_vegan

www.facebook.com/Dilliciously-Vegan

Follow My Cafe

https://www.instagram.com/hungrycatcafe1

CONTENTS

Introduction

My journey to veganism began 8 years ago when I made a conscious decision to commit to values which had become intrinsic in my life. Respecting the earth and every life birthed into it. Being vegan works well for the lifestyle I have adopted. Trying to live simply, enjoying what each day has to offer and to be thankful for being alive! Being conscious about each decision you make and taking responsibility for your actions in this journey called life, respecting each other and every being, has centred me and reconnected me to the world.

I grew up in a family that enjoys food and celebration, so to me every meal is special and built on memories. Many of my recipes are adaptions from my grandmother and mother who are both phenomenal cooks. My many years of experience in catering and hospitality have also helped me to perfect the dishes. The root of my food is Greek in origin as this is my heritage - flavoursome, varied and exciting!

So after travelling to different parts of the world and touring England with a catering van visiting festivals, I decided to be stationary for bit, set up a vegan cafe and decided to write this cookbook of my recipes. I hope you find as much enjoyment in preparing these dishes at home as I have had serving to thousands of happy customers over the years. It gives me great joy when non-vegans try my food, it is a point of engagement and education. We all have something to learn and much to improve on.

This cookbook is a collection of meals for the family, dishes to impress, comfort food and a vegan take on signature stables. Weather you prefer savoury or sweet, it meets all tastes. I've tried to present it in a simple and easy step by step guide, suitable even for the beginner cook.

Enjoy and please let me know what you think!

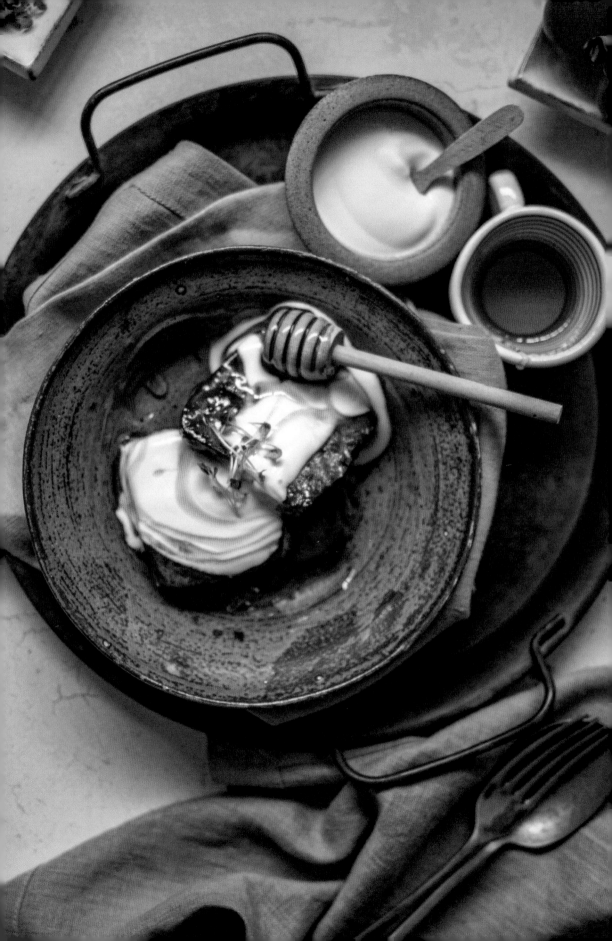

Breakfast

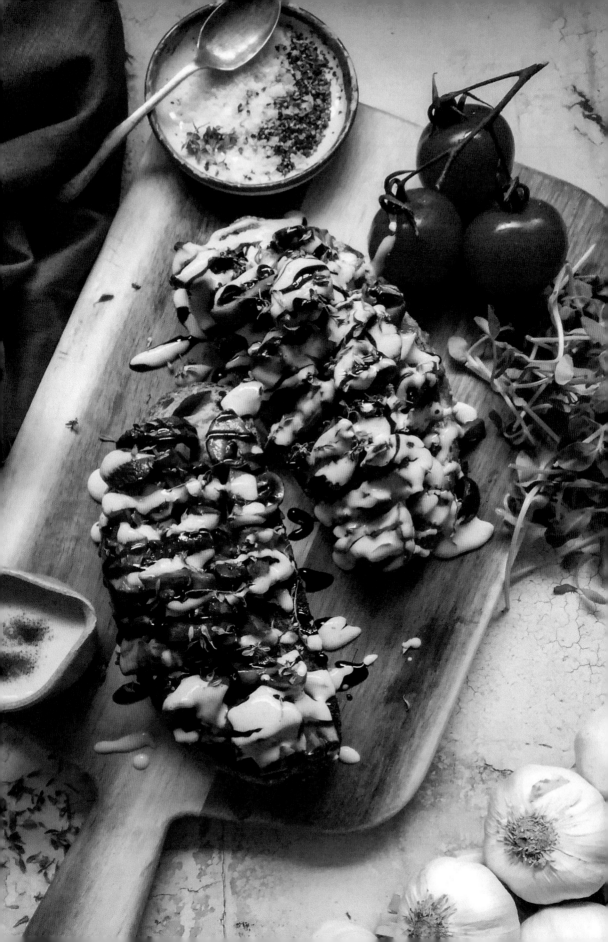

Garlic Mushrooms on Toast with Cheese Sauce

Serve: 2

Ingredients

- Fresh Artisan Bread of your choice
- 250-300g Chestnut or Portobello Mushrooms quartered / sliced
- 3- 4 Garlic cloves finely chopped
- 2 Tbsp Olive Oil
- Finely chopped Parsley to garnish
- Balsamic Glaze to drizzle over

For The Cheese Sauce

- 1 Tbsp Plain Flour
- 2 Tbsp Olive Oil
- ½ Tsp Smoked Paprika
- 1 Cup Soya Milk
- ½ Tsp English mustard
- 1-2 Tbsp Nutritional Yeast (Optional)
- ½ - 1 tsp turmeric powder to make a nice cheese colour
- Salt & Pepper to taste

Method

1. First make the cheese sauce. Put the oil into a non stick pan, med- to high heat. When the oil has heated add the flour and stir, it will turn into a paste. Start adding the milk bit by bit and mix well. Once you've added all the milk, simmer to med heat. If you have any lumps, this happens if you add all the milk at once, use a whisk and stir vigorously to get rid of the lumps. Now add the rest of the ingredients in and stir well, taste and season. Simmer for 5 minutes and the sauce will be ready. If it hasn't thickened enough leave it on simmer for a few more minutes. Set aside to drizzle over the mushrooms. You can reheat the sauce if needed.

2. Put the oil & mushrooms in a pan, med – high heat and cook for about 5 minutes, you want some of the mushrooms liquid left in the pan. Now add the garlic and cook for another minute or until there is no more liquid left. Toast your bread just before the mushrooms are done, place the mushrooms on the toast, drizzle with cheese sauce then drizzle with balsamic and garnish with the parsley.

TIP:
You could have this for breakfast, brunch or lunch. Serve with a nice fresh salad to balance it out.

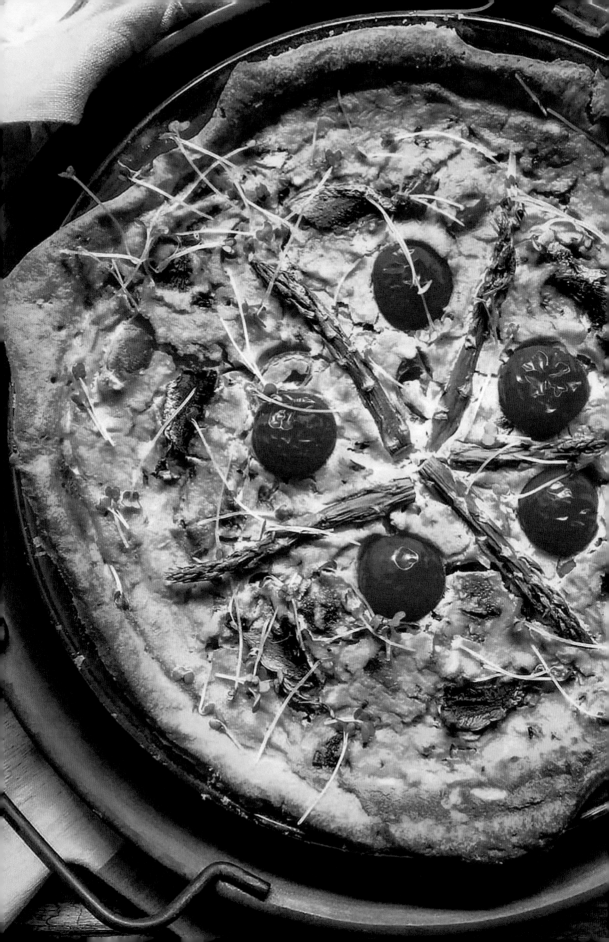

Mushroom, Asparagus & Cherry Tomato Quiche

Serves 4 – 6

It's the first time I ever made a quiche and am very happy with the results and how easy it is to make. You can experiment with all sorts of vegetables and create your own masterpiece. I used these ingredients as I think they go very well together.

Ingredients

- 375g Short crust pastry at room temperature.
- 400g Firm Tofu
- 50g Cashew Nuts
- 20g Nutritional Yeast (Optional)
- 160ml Soya Cream
- 1 Tsp Turmeric Powder
- Salt & Pepper to taste
- 100g Mushrooms of your choice sliced
- 100g Asparagus chopped, keep tips for the top to decorate
- 100g Cherry Tomatoes halved
- Cheese of choice (Optional) You can add into the mix or sprinkle on top before baking. I didn't use cheese.

Method

1. Preheat the oven 190 fan or 170 conventional ovens. Grease a 9" pan and place your pastry in it, no need to blind bake. Make holes in the pastry using a fork so the steam can escape. Bake for 10 minutes or until light brown in colour.

2. While that is baking, put all ingredients, except the vegetables in a food processor and mix till you have a nice smooth texture. Remove from the processor and transfer into a bowl and then mix your vegetables in using a spatula. Remember to keep some vegetables aside to decorate the top of the quiche.

3. Pour the mixture into the baked pastry and level it out with a spatula. Now you can decorate the top with vegetables, if you using cheese sprinkle it on before you decorate.

4. Turn your oven down to 180 fan or 160 conventional and bake for a further 30 to 40 minutes or when its golden brown. Mine was done in 30 minutes.

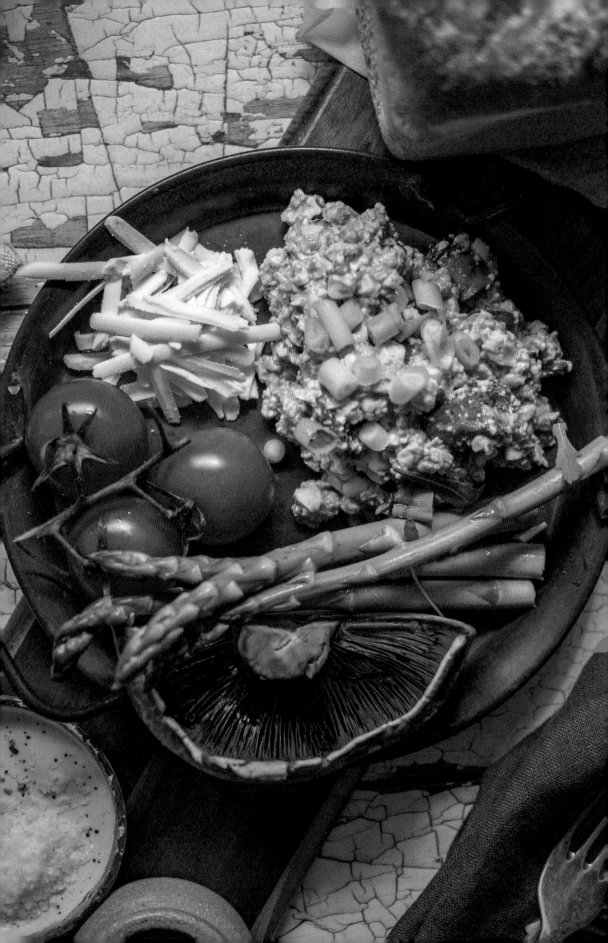

Scrambled Tofu with Mushrooms & Cheese

Serves 2

I really used to love eating scrambled eggs with cheese and mushrooms and I'm so glad that Tofu is such a great substitute for scrambled eggs. Like many, it took me a while to experiment with tofu as I thought it was a tasteless ingredient, luckily I continued to try it in different ways and absolutely love it now that I know how to cook it! Keep trying and experimenting and you will see how easy & tasty it is and of course very good for you, packed with protein.

Ingredients

- 349g Silken Tofu (Firm tofu will also do)
- 1 Tsp Turmeric Powder
- 1 Tbsp Olive Oil
- 2 Portobello Mushrooms Sliced
- Handful of grated Cheddar Cheese
- Salt & Pepper to taste
- Nutritional Yeast (Optional) adds a nutty and cheesy flavour.
- 2 Spring onions finely chopped (optional) to garnish the dish when serving.

Method

1. In a pan on a med to high heat put the oil and mushrooms & cook for about 3 minutes.

2. Then add the tofu, using a wooden spoon or fork to break up the tofu until it looks scrambled, add the turmeric, salt & pepper and cook for a further 5 minutes. Turn off the heat and stir in the cheese and nutritional yeast if using. Taste to see if you need more seasoning. Enjoy xx

3. Serve on toast or add to a full breakfast.

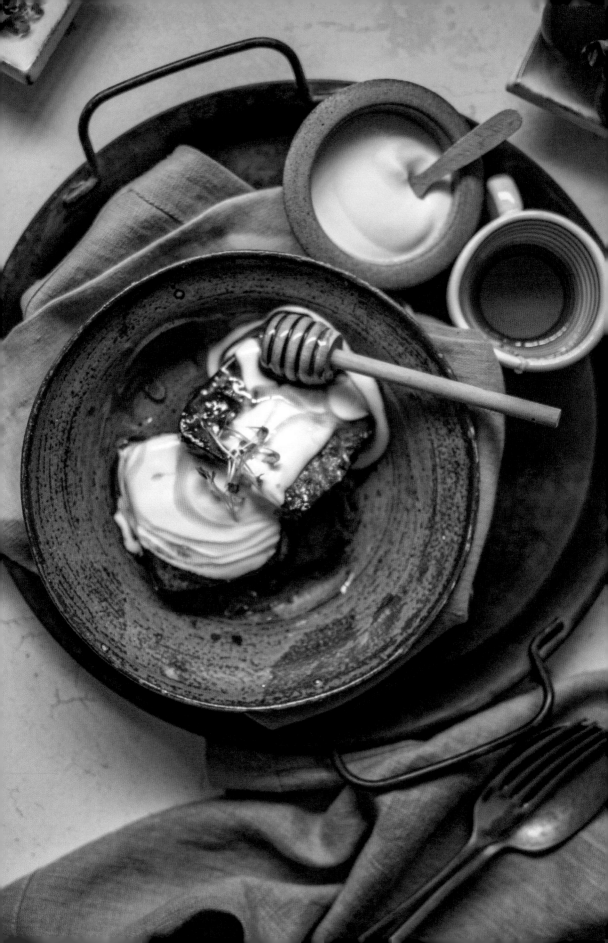

Sweet & Sour Tofu with Pecan Nuts, Yogurt & Syrup

Serves 2

This recipe came about when I had a craving for something both sweet and savoury. I absolutely love it and its one of my favourite recipes. It's so easy & quick to make. I hope you enjoy it as much as I do x

Ingredients

- 350 -400 g Firm Tofu
- 2-4 tbsp Maple or Golden Syrup
- 2-4 tbsp Soy Yogurt
- Pecan or Mixed Nuts to sprinkle on to

Marinade

- 1 Tbsp Dark Soy Sauce
- 2 Tbsp Bbq Sauce
- 2 Tbsp Vegetable Oil

Method

1. Mix marinade ingredient into a bowl/ plate. Cut tofu into 1-2cm thick slices. Place the tofu into the marinade, turn over so all sides are coated with the marinade.

2. In a non-stick pan on med to high heat, place the tofu in the pan and cook for 2 min on each side. You can dip the cooked tofu in the left over marinade before dressing with remainder ingredients.

3. Plate up the tofu, then put a dollop of yogurt, drizzle with syrup and sprinkle the nuts on top.

4. You can have this for breakfast, lunch or for when you feel like something sweet.

TIP:

You can make extra marinade to have at hand for your next tofu recipe and keep it in a bottle in the fridge for a long while. If you new to tofu and want more flavour in your tofu dishes, let the tofu marinade overnight as tofu absorbs any flavour you add to it and the longer you leave it in the marinade, the more flavour it will absorb.

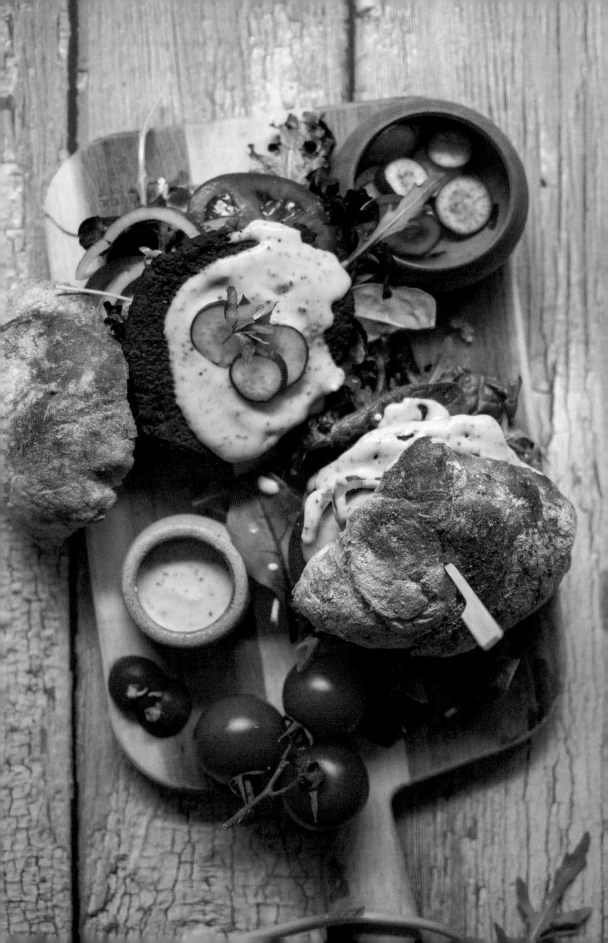

Burgers

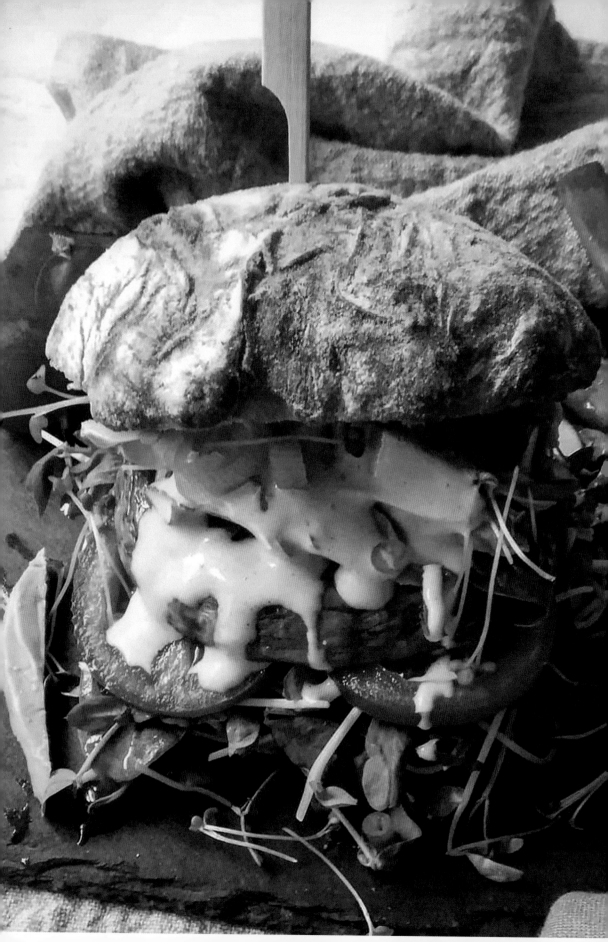

Mushroom, Avocado & Cheese Sauce Burger

Serves 1

Ingredients

- 1 Burger Bun
- ½ Avocado sliced
- 1 Large Portobello Mushroom, stalk removed

For dressing burger bun

- Some Mixed Salad leaves, pea shoots, & cress sprouts
- 1 Spring Onion finely sliced
- 1 Radish finely sliced
- 2 slices Tomato

Cheese Sauce serves: 2-3

- 1 Tbsp Plain Flour
- 1 & ½ Tbsp Olive Oil
- Salt & Pepper to taste
- ½ Tsp Smoked Paprika
- 1 Cup Plant Milk plus extra if needed
- ½ tsp English mustard
- ½ - 1 tsp turmeric powder for colour
- 1-2 tbsp nutritional yeast optional for a nutty & cheesy flavour

Method

1. Start by making the cheese sauce as you can reheat it if needed. In a pan, heat up the olive oil on a med-high heat. Add the flour and stir; it will turn into a yellow paste. Pour the milk in bit by bit stirring after each pour to avoid lumps. Once all the milk has been used up, simmer and add the remainder ingredients and keep stirring every minute or so, it will start to thicken. If you have lumps in the sauce, use a hand whisk and stir vigorously to get rid of the lumps. You can also use a hand blender to remove lumps and also get a smoother sauce. If the sauce is too thick you can add some extra milk.

2. Add a drop of oil in a pan on a med – high heat and cook the mushroom whole for 3-5 minutes each side. Start to dress your bun. Start with a drizzle of cheese sauce then add mixed leaves & tomato. On top of that put the cooked mushroom, salad leaves, avocado slices, cheese sauce, pea shoots, sprouts, onions and radishes.

3. Tip, to keep your avocado form turning brown, drizzle some lemon or lime over it.

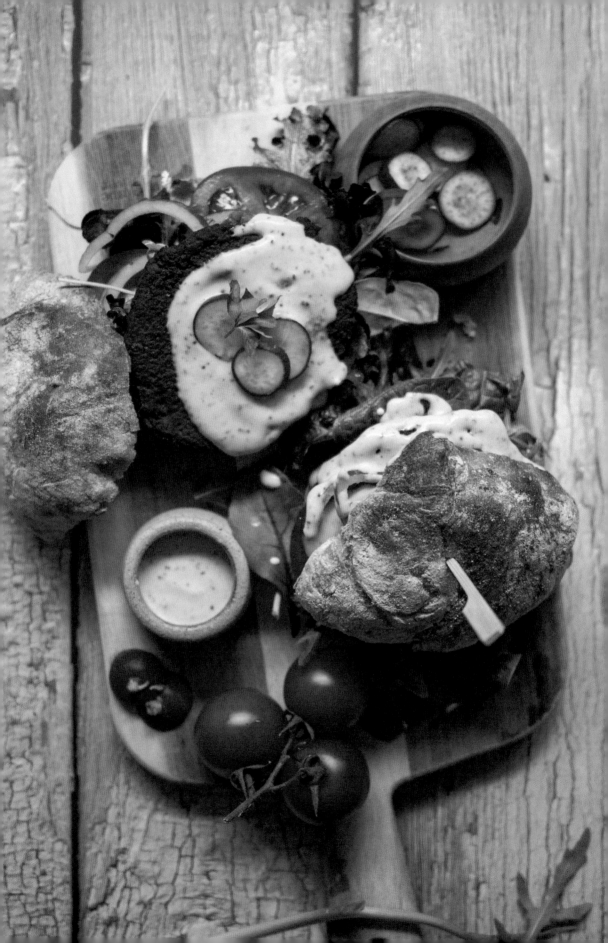

Beetroot & Mustard Sauce Burger

Serves 6-8

Ingredients

- 600g raw beetroot quartered
- 1 Cup Chickpea Flour
- 2 Garlic cloves
- 1 Red Onion Quartered
- 1Tsp Salt
- 1 Tsp Pepper
- 1 Tsp Smoked Paprika
- 1 Tin 400g chickpeas, drained
- 1 Tbsp dried parsley
- ½ Tsp Olive Oil
- 1-2 Tbsp Plain Flour (if needed)
- **Yogurt Dressing**
- 1 Cup Soya Yogurt
- 1 Tsp English mustard
- 1 Tsp Wholegrain mustard
- Salt & Pepper to taste
- **Burger Dressing**
- Mixed leaf salad
- Tomato
- Red Onion
- Rocket leaves
- Radish

Method

1. In a non-stick pan on a med heat put the chickpea flour and stir continuously for about 5 minutes, it will start giving off a nutty smell, keep stirring or it will burn. Stir for a further 2 minutes and remove from the heat to cool. Once the chickpea flour cools down, put all the ingredients in a food processor except the oil and plain flour. Process till everything is mixed well and finely chopped. If the mixture seems to dry, add the oil and mix again. Transfer mixture to a bowl and start shaping. Make a ball in the palm of your hand and flatten to form a patty shape. If the mixture seems to wet you can add some of the plain flour and mix well. You shouldn't need more than 2 Tbsp of plain flour.

2. Make the yogurt dressing. In a bowl mix all the dressing ingredients together and set aside.

3. Toast buns and set aside. In a non-stick pan on a med -high heat, cook the beetroot patties about 3 minutes each side.

4. Dress your buns. Start with a drizzle of yogurt dressing, then salad leaves, tomatoes and onions. Now add the beetroot patty, drizzle more dressing and top with more salad leaves, rocket and radishes and a final drizzle of dressing,

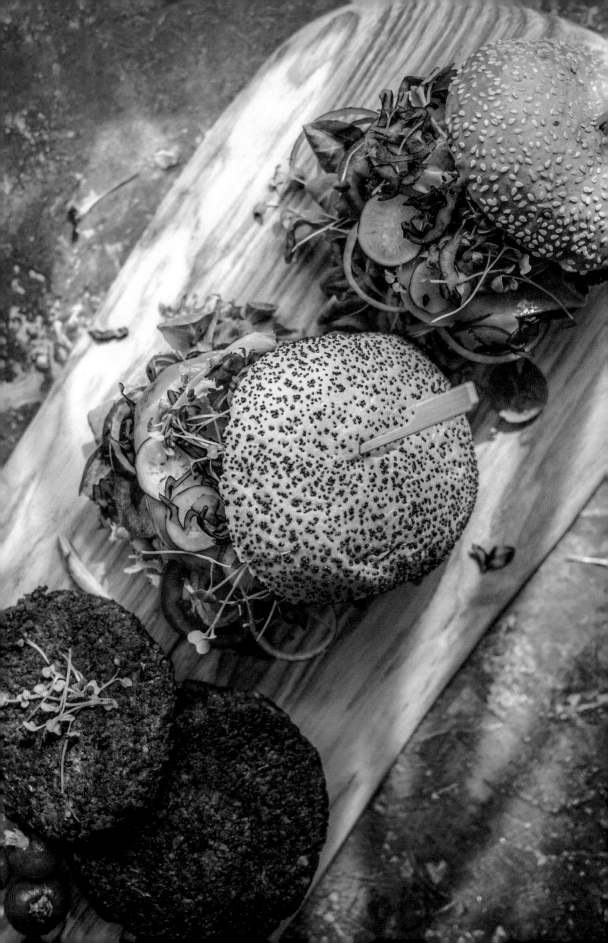

Black Bean & Lentil Burger Patties

Serves 4-6

With this recipe, I tried to recreate the flavours of my mother's meatballs I used to have as a child. The thing I liked most about them was that I could taste the green peppers and onions so I added those two ingredients in this recipe to share that wonderful memory of flavour with you...

I dressed my burgers with mixed leaf salad, tomatoes, onions, cheese, radishes, watercress, red cabbage, chilli mayo and plain mayonnaise.

Ingredients

- 400g (1 tin) Drained Black lentils (any lentils if you can't find black)
- 400g (1 tin) Drained Black beans
- 1 Green Pepper diced
- ½ Red Onion diced
- 250g breadcrumbs
- 3 Sprigs Parsley
- 1 Garlic clove roughly chopped
- Salt & pepper to taste
- Vegetable oil for pan frying

Method

1. Put all ingredients into a food processor and mix till everything has combined well.

2. Don't over mix so you have a nice texture and bite. Taste and season, remove from the processor and transfer into a bowl.

3. Lightly oil a non stick pan, med – high heat. Take a handful of the mixture, forming a ball in your hands then flatten and shape.

4. Pan Fry 2-3 minutes on each side or till lightly browned.

TIP:

You can also make meat balls with this, using smaller amounts of mixture and pan fry or deep fry. Once you've made them they can last in the fridge for 4 - 5days. They also freeze well.

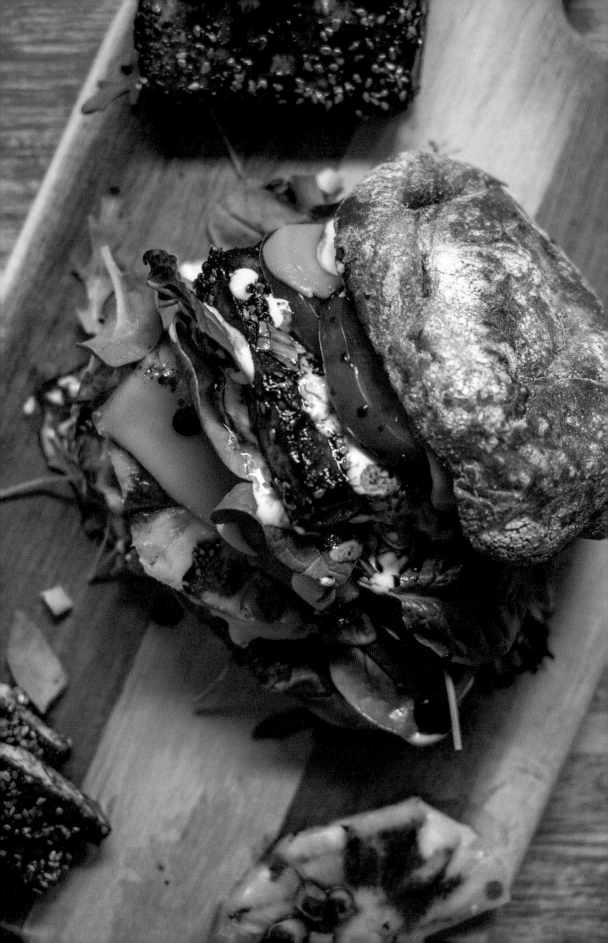

Tofu, Pineapple and Cheese Burger

Serves 1

Ingredients

- 1 Burger bun Toasted
- 1 Thick 2-4cm Slice of firm Tofu
- 2 Slices Cheddar Cheese
- 1 Thick Slice Fresh pineapple
- Mixed salad leaves
- 1 Spring Onion Finely Chopped or Red onion if you prefer
- 2 Slices Tomato
- Mayonnaise
- Marinade
- 1 Tbsp Dark Soya Sauce
- 1 Tsp vegetable oil
- Sesame seeds

Method

1. Mix the marinade ingredients together and fully coat the tofu steak, leave it in the marinade till you ready to pan fry it. If you want it to absorb more flavour, marinade it overnight. Toast bun and set aside.

2. Get all your salad prepped and ready to dress your bun. Drizzle some mayonnaise at the bottom of the bun, then add salad leaves, tomato, pineapple, a slice of cheese and drizzle more mayonnaise.

3. On a med-high heat in a non stick pan, pan fry the tofu for 2-3 min on each side, when you've turned it over add the other slice of cheese on top of the tofu so it can melt.

4. Remove from the heat and place on the dressed bun. Add more salad leaves, tomato and onions.

5. Drizzle again with mayonnaise and the remaining marinade.

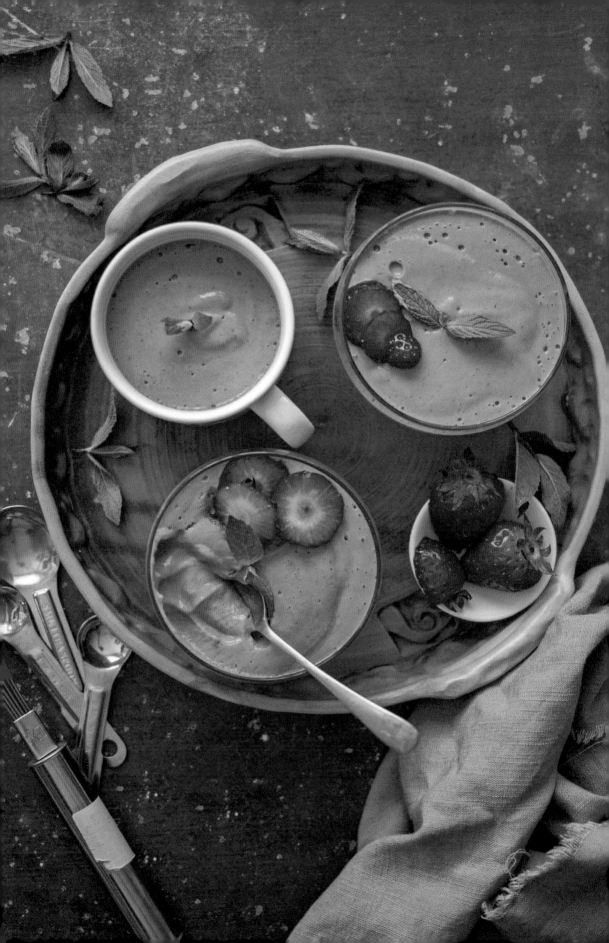

Cakes

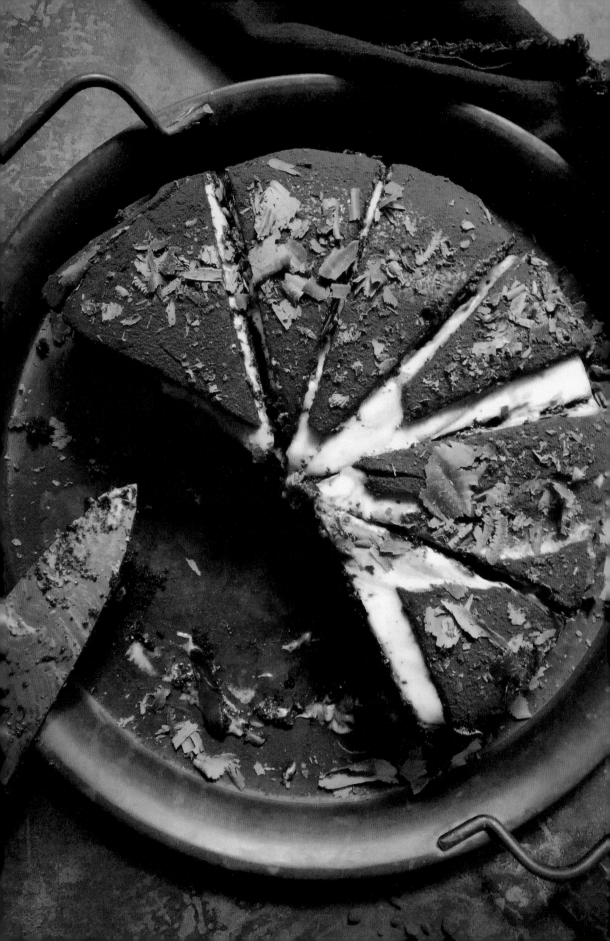

Chocolate Mocha with chocolate Ganache

 8-10- Slices

Ingredients

Cake Mix
- 250g Self Rising Flour
- 50g Cacao Powder
- 1 Tsp Ground Coffee
- 1 Tsp Bicarbonate of soda
- 300ml Soya Milk
- 1 Tbsp Apple Cider Vinegar
- 150g Plant margarine at

room temperature
- ½ Tsp Salt
- 200g Caster Sugar
- ½ Tsp vanilla essence

Frosting
- 310g icing sugar
- 75g Lotus Biscoff spread
- 1 Tsp Vanilla essence

- 3-4 Tbsp Milk

Ganache
- 100g of 70% or more dark chocolate finely chopped
- 100g soy milk
- Chocolate shavings to decorate
- Cacao Powder to decorate

Method

1. Preheat oven at 160 Fan or 180 Conventional ovens.
2. Grease, line and sprinkle with flour, 1x 8 "bake tin.
3. Put the milk and cider vinegar in a jug and set aside.
4. Sift the flour, cacao, coffee and bicarbonate into a bowl and set aside.
5. In a large mixing bowl, put the margarine, salt, sugar and vanilla and mix with a hand mixer on high speed until the mixture is fluffy and pale in colour, this can take 6-8 minutes.
6. Now you going to mix the rest of the ingredients into the large bowl, alternating the flour and liquid.
7. Start adding some of the flour to the butter mix whilst still mixing the butter mix with the hand mixer. If using a stand mixer leave it on whilst adding the ingredients to it. You start with adding the flour and end with adding the flour. (Flour, liquid, flour, liquid, flour)
8. Once you've added the first bit of flour, whilst mixing, mix till combined then add half of the liquid mixture till combined then add more flour, combine then remainder of the liquid, combine and the remainder flour and combine.. Once this is done use a spatula and go round the sides of the bowl making sure everything is mixed in and well combined. You should have an airy and smooth cake mixture.
9. Pour the cake mixture into the cake tin and bake for 45-55 minutes. Check it after 45 minutes by inserting a wooden skewer in the middle to see if it comes out dry, if not it needs more baking. Sometimes you can see before taking it out of the oven, that it's not ready, the centre will seem like it's still raw, in this case don't remove from the oven and close the oven door quickly so as not to lose too much heat. I would suggest checking it

again after 10 minutes before taking it out and doing the skewer test. Once it's done remove from the oven and let it sit in the tin for 10 minutes before transferring it onto a cooling rack. Once cooled cut the cake in half and let it cool further.

10. Mix the frosting ingredients together but don't add all the milk at once add it bit by bit whilst mixing with a hand mixer. You want the frosting to be a bit thicker than usual as you going to pour ganache over it. To frost the middle of the cake take some of the frosting, enough to frost the middle and add a little milk to it so its easer to spread.

11. Place the bottom half of the cake on a stand and frost, then place the top half on and frost the entire cake. You don't want a thick layer of frosting on the entire cake especially the top as you still need to pour the ganache over the frosting so it's better to have a thin layer of frosting. When done put the cake in the fridge for an hour so the frosting can set. Take the cake out after an hour and stat on the ganache.

12. Roughly chop the chocolate into small pieces or use a food processor and pulse. You don't want to have any big pieces of chocolate. Transfer the chocolate to a heat proof bowl and set aside. Your dark chocolate must be 70% or more or it will split.

13. In a wide pan on a med –low heat add the milk and keep an eye on it, you want it to get to the point before it boils. When you see the steam rising it's time to remove from the heat and pour over the chocolate. Do not stir, let it sit for about 30-40 seconds then use a spatula and stir it until it turns into a glossy ganache. I would leave it for 5 minutes before pouring over the cake. Sprinkle some cacao powder and chocolate shavings over the top and let it set in the fridge for an hour.

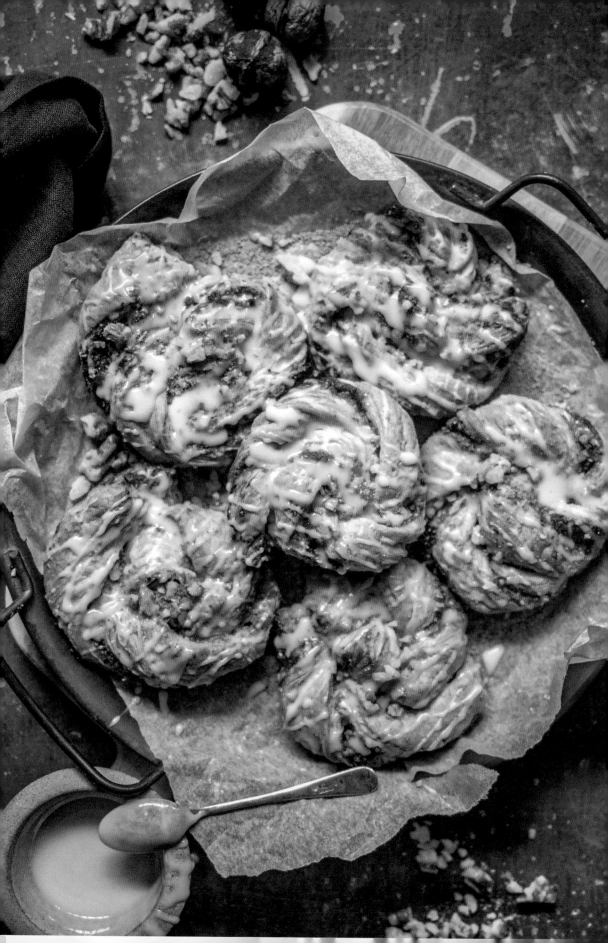

Cinnamon Buns with Pecan Nuts

Makes 6-8

Ingredients

- 2 x 375g Puff pastry
- ½ cup brown sugar
- 2Tbsp Ground Cinnamon
- 2 Tbsp melted and cooled margarine/butter
- Handful of chopped pecan nuts

Glaze

- ½ cup icing sugar
- 1 Tbsp water

Method

1. Preheat the oven to 200 fan or 220 conventional ovens.
2. Grease a 16x12" baking pan. Your baking pan needs to be large enough to allow the pastry to expand and make sure you space them out on the baking tray.
3. Unroll 1 of the pastries and brush it with the melted butter.
4. Mix the sugar and cinnamon together and sprinkle on top of the butter. You can add some nuts here too.
5. Now take the second pastry and cover the one with the filling, press it down lightly especially around the edges so it sticks together.
6. Now cut the pastry, vertically or horizontally, whichever you prefer. The difference will be larger or smaller buns when done. Whichever way you choose to cut it, start by cutting it in half, then half the half and so on or you could measure it and cut the strips that way. An ideal width would be 2-4cm.
7. Once you've cut your strips, take one, hold one end and start to twist it, not too tight and not too lose. Once twisted, start to roll it whilst it's flat on the surface till the end to form the bun shape. Tuck & pinch the lose end under the rolled up bun so it keeps its shape whilst baking.
8. Place them on the baking tray leaving enough room between them to expand.
9. Bake for 15-20 minutes or till golden brown.
10. Transfer to a cooling rack and allow cooling for 5-10 minutes before glazing.
11. Mix the glaze ingredients till you have a thick, pourable consistency.
12. Using a spoon, drizzle the glaze over the buns and sprinkle with nuts

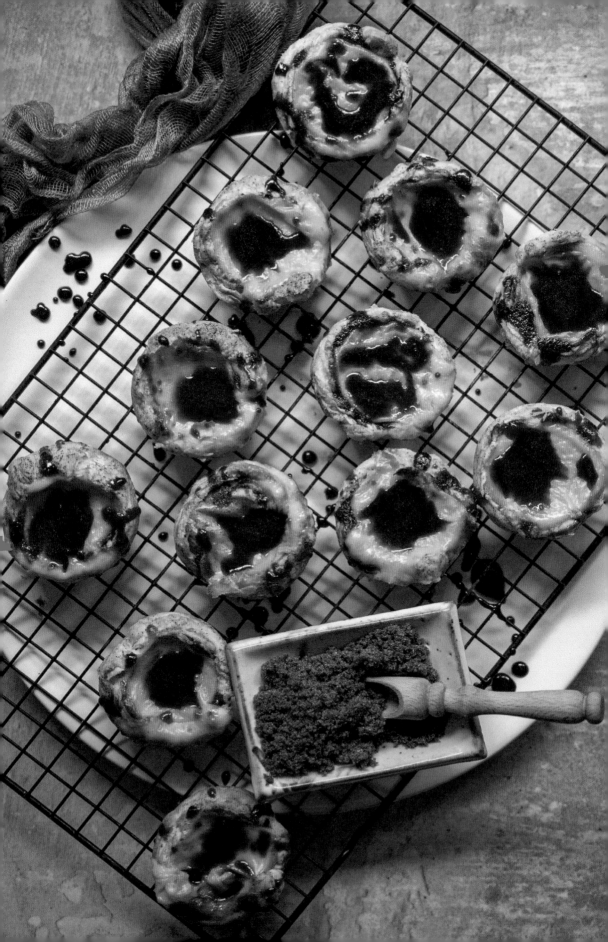

Portuguese Custard Tarts

 Makes 12

Ingredients

- 1 x 375g puff pastry at room temperature
- 2-3 Tbsp ground cinnamon
- 400 ml Soya milk
- 3 Tbsp Custard Powder
- 3 Tbsp Sugar

Caramel topping
- 75g muscovado sugar
- 1 Tbsp water

Method

1. Take a cup out of the 400ml milk and aside to mix the custard powder in

2. In a med sized pan, on a high heat, bring the rest of the milk to the boil, add the sugar in at the same time and stir till the sugar has dissolved.

3. Mix the custard power into the cup of milk and stir well till it all turns to liquid without any lumps.

4. When the milk comes to the boil, simmer and add the custard milk into the pan and immediately stir it in and keep stirring to avoid lumps and burning. If you do get lumps, use a whisk or hand blender to get rid of the lumps. Keep stirring for 5 minutes, it will thicken.

5. Remove from the heat and let it cool down (You could make it the day before and whisk it smooth when you need it)

6. Preheat the oven to 200 fan or 220 conventional ovens

7. Lay your pastry out on a flat surface lengthways.

8. Sprinkle the cinnamon all over it and rub it in with your hands.

9. Start rolling the pastry lengthways away from you as if making a Swiss roll, When you get to the end, turn the pastry so the fold is underneath.

10. To cut the pastry, either measure it and cut it into 12 pieces or cut it in half, then half that half and so on until you have 12 pieces. You looking at about 2cm or so width per piece.

11. Grease a muffin tray

12. Take one of your cut pieces and turn it so that the spiral is facing upwards, using the palm of your hand flatten the pastry, repeat for the remaining 11 pieces. Once this is done take one flattened piece and put it into the muffin tray. Using your fingers start to press the pastry outwards so it goes up the sides, like hollow cups to fill with the custard later. When this is done with the rest of them place it in the oven on the top shelf and bake for 8-10 minutes or until golden and puffed up.

13. Take them out the oven and use a teaspoon to push the parts that have puffed up so you have space for the custard. The custard should be cooled before filling but not essential.

14. Fill the pasty with custard but don't overfill as it will overflow when baking. When they all filled place them back in the oven, again on the top shelf and bake for a further 10 minutes or nice and golden

15. Remove from the oven, using a butter knife, go round the edges of the tarts to release them from the pan and use a teaspoon to lift them out and transfer onto a cooling rack.

16. Now make the caramel, this cannot be done before hand. In a small pan on a high heat add the mascovado sugar and leave it for 30 seconds or so then add the water and leave it on a high heat until it turns into lava, do not stir it. When it's bubbling like lava it's done, this happens very quickly, it's ready in a minute or so. Be careful as this is very hot and dangerous.

17. Remove from the heat and use a tablespoon to pour the caramel over the tarts. Let them cool before trying.

18. Place the caramel pan in cold water immediately

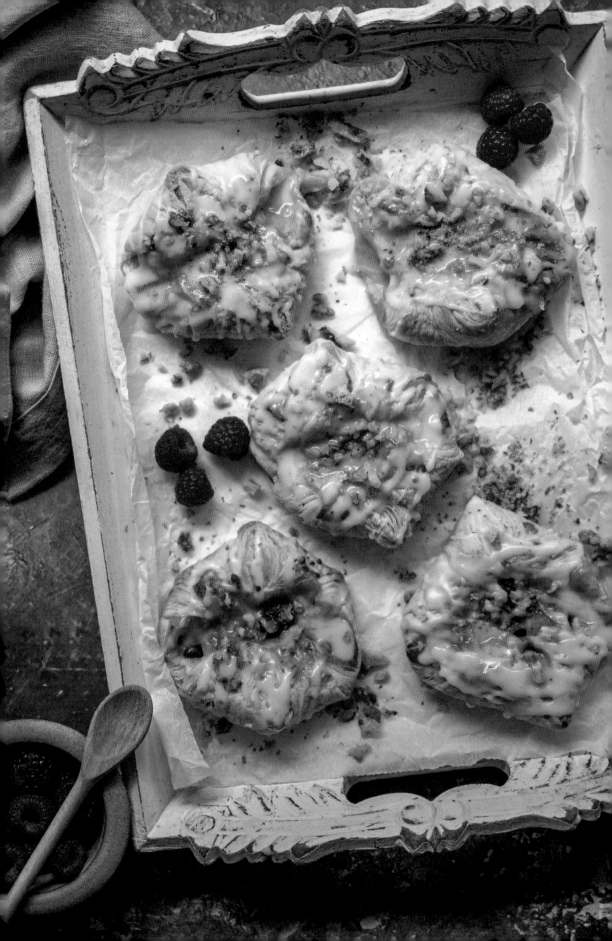

Danish Custard, Pecan & Raspberry Pastries

 Makes 8

With this recipe I made half plain custard and nuts and half custard, raspberries and nuts. If you want to only make the raspberries then double up on the raspberries or if you only want to make the nuts version, double up on the nuts.

Ingredients

- 1 pack 375g Puff Pastry room temperature
- 250ml Soya Milk
- 2 Tbsp Custard Powder
- 2 Tbsp Sugar
- Handful of pecan Nuts roughly chopped
- Handful of Raspberries
- Glaze
- ½ Cup Icing Sugar
- 1 Tbsp Water

Method

1. Preheat oven to 200 Fan or 220 conventional Ovens

2. Make the custard first. Take 4 Tbsp of the 250ml milk and put it in a cup, add the custard powder into the cup and stir until its all liquid without any lumps. Set it aside but give it a stir again before the milk in the pan boils.

3. In a med size pan on a high heat add the sugar, the rest of the milk and bring to the boil, stir to dissolve the sugar. When the milk starts to boil, pour the custard milk into the pan whilst stirring to avoid lumps, simmer immediately and keep stirring for about 3-5 minutes. The custard will thicken. If you get lumps remove them by using a hand blender or whisk. Set aside to cool. It can thicken more when cooling, if so just whisk again when you ready to use it.

4. Lay your pastry out flat on a surface. You can make 4 or 8 pastries. Either cut the pastry into 8 squares for smaller pastries or 4 squares for larger ones.

5. Place the squares on a greased baking pan, layer each square with custard 1-2 Tbsp for the larger one and ½ - 1 Tbsp for the smaller ones. If you making the raspberry pastries, add 2-4 raspberries depending on square size and nuts if you like. For the plain custard add some nuts on top of the custard.

6. To fold the pastry, take the opposite corners and bring them together and do the same for all 4 corners. When you have all the corners together, pinch them together and push them into the centre of the pastry so they keep their shape whilst baking.(Like folding each corner into the centre and pressing to secure)

7. When they folded and pressed, put a dollop of custard on top of the pressed down centre and sprinkle with nuts and raspberries.

8. Bake at the bottom of the oven for 20-30 minutes or until golden.

9. Remove from the oven and transfer to a cooling rack. Let them cool down before glazing as the glaze will melt.

10. For the glaze mix the icing sugar and water together, you need a thick but pourable consistency, add more water or icing sugar as needed.

11. Using a spoon, drizzle the glaze over the pastries and add more nuts if you like.

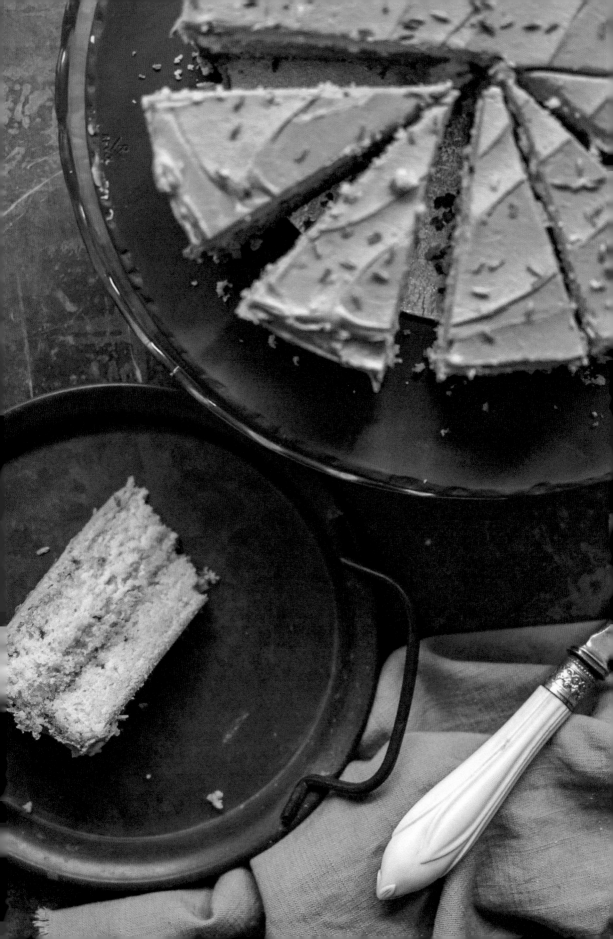

Lavender Cake

 10-12 Slices

Ingredients

- Cake Mix
- 300g Self Rising Flour
- 1 Tsp Bicarbonate of soda
- 1 Tbsp Dried edible lavender
- 300ml Soya Milk
- 1 Tbsp Apple Cider Vinegar
- 150g Plant margarine at room temperature
- ½ Tsp Salt
- 200g Caster Sugar
- ½ Tsp vanilla essence
- Frosting
- 450g Icing Sugar
- 45g Butter
- 1 Tsp Vanilla Essence
- 4 Tbsp Soya Milk (Added bit by bit)
- Purple / Lilac food Colouring
- Decorate / topping
- ½-1 Tbsp dry edible lavender

Method

1. Preheat oven at 160 Fan or 180 Conventional ovens.
2. Grease, line and sprinkle with flour, 1 x 8 "bake tin.
3. Put the milk and cider vinegar in a jug and set aside.
4. Sift the flour and bicarbonate into a bowl, add the lavender and set aside.
5. In a large mixing bowl, put the margarine, salt, sugar and vanilla and mix with a hand mixer on high speed until the mixture is fluffy and pale in colour, this can take 6-8 minutes.
6. Now you going to mix the rest of the ingredients into the large bowl, alternating the flour and liquid.
7. Start adding some of the flour to the butter mix whilst still mixing the butter mix with the hand mixer. If using a stand mixer leave it on whilst adding the ingredients to it. You start with adding the flour and end with adding the flour. (Flour, liquid, flour, liquid, flour)
8. Once you've added the first bit of flour, whilst mixing, mix till combined then add half of the liquid mixture till combined then add more flour, combine then remainder of the liquid, combine and the remainder flour and combine.. Once this is done use a spatula and go round the sides of the bowl making sure everything is mixed in and well combined. You should have an airy and smooth cake mixture.
9. Pour the cake mixture into the cake tin and bake for 45-55 minutes. Check it after 45 minutes by inserting a wooden skewer in the middle to see if it comes out dry, if not it needs more baking. Sometimes you can see before taking it out of the oven, that it's not ready, the centre will seem like it's still raw, in this case don't remove from the oven and close the oven door quickly so as not to lose too much heat. I would suggest checking it again after 10 minutes before taking it out and doing the skewer test. Once it's done remove from the oven and let it sit in the tin for 10 minutes before transferring it onto a cooling rack.
10. When the cake has cooled down, cut the cake in half so you can add frosting in the middle of the cake, it will need to cool further once cut.
11. Using a hand mixer, mix the frosting ingredients together but not all the milk, start with 2 Tbsp and add the rest if needed. Add the food colouring bit by bit whilst mixing till you get the desired colour.
12. When the cake has cooled down, place the bottom half on a cake stand and use a cake spatula to frost it. Then sandwich the top to the bottom and frost the entire cake. Sprinkle with lavender

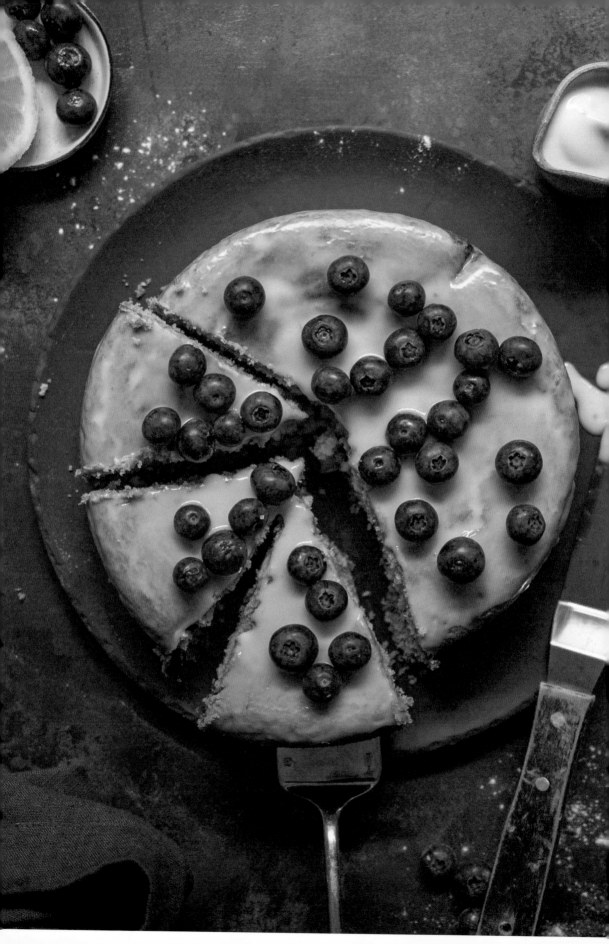

Blueberry & Lemon Cake

 10-12 Slices

Ingredients

Cake Mix

- 300g Self Rising Flour
- 1 Tsp Bicarbonate of soda
- 200ml Soya Milk
- 1 Tbsp Apple Cider Vinegar
- 150g Plant margarine at room temperature
- ½ Tsp Salt
- 200g Caster Sugar
- ½ Tsp vanilla essence
- Zest of 2 large Lemons
- 122g fresh blueberries (using half at a time)

Icing

- 1Cup Icing Sugar
- Juice of 1 lemon
- Milk if needed
- Fresh blueberries to decorate

Method

1. Preheat oven at 160 Fan or 180 Conventional ovens.
2. Grease, line and sprinkle with flour, 1x 8 "bake tin.
3. Put the milk and cider vinegar in a jug and set aside.
4. Sift the flour and bicarbonate into a bowl and set aside.
5. In a large mixing bowl, put the margarine, salt, sugar, lemon zest and vanilla and mix with a hand mixer on high speed until the mixture is fluffy and pale in colour, this can take 6-8 minutes.
6. Now you going to mix the rest of the ingredients, except the blueberries, into the large bowl, alternating the flour and liquid.
7. Start adding some of the flour to the butter mix whilst still mixing the butter mix with the hand mixer. If using a stand mixer leave it on whilst adding the ingredients to it. You start with adding the flour and end with adding the flour. (Flour, liquid, flour, liquid, flour)
8. Once you've added the first bit of flour, whilst mixing, mix till combined then add half of the liquid mixture till combined then add more flour, combine then remainder of the liquid, combine and the remainder flour and combine.. Once this is done use a spatula and go round the sides of the bowl making sure everything is mixed in and well combined. You should have an airy and smooth cake mixture. Fold in half of the fresh blueberries.
9. Pour the cake mixture into the cake tin and put the other half of the blueberries in now without stirring, just sprinkle them over the top once the cake mix is in the baking tin and bake for 45-55 minutes. Check it after 45 minutes by inserting a wooden skewer in the middle to see if it comes out dry, if not it needs more baking. Sometimes you can see before taking it out of the oven, that it's not ready, the centre will seem like it's still raw, in this case don't remove from the oven and close the oven door quickly so as not to lose too much heat. I would suggest checking it again after 10 minutes before taking it out and doing the skewer test. Once it's done remove from the oven and let it sit in the tin for 10 minutes before transferring it onto a cooling rack.
10. Make the Icing when the cake has cooled down by mixing the frosting ingredients together. It should be a thick pourable consistency. You can add some milk if it's too thick or more icing sugar if too runny.
11. Once the cake has cooled down completely, transfer it to a cake stand and pour the icing over the cake by starting in the centre and using a spatula to spread the icing all over the cake, push the icing to the edges so it can run down the sides. Decorate with fresh blueberries.

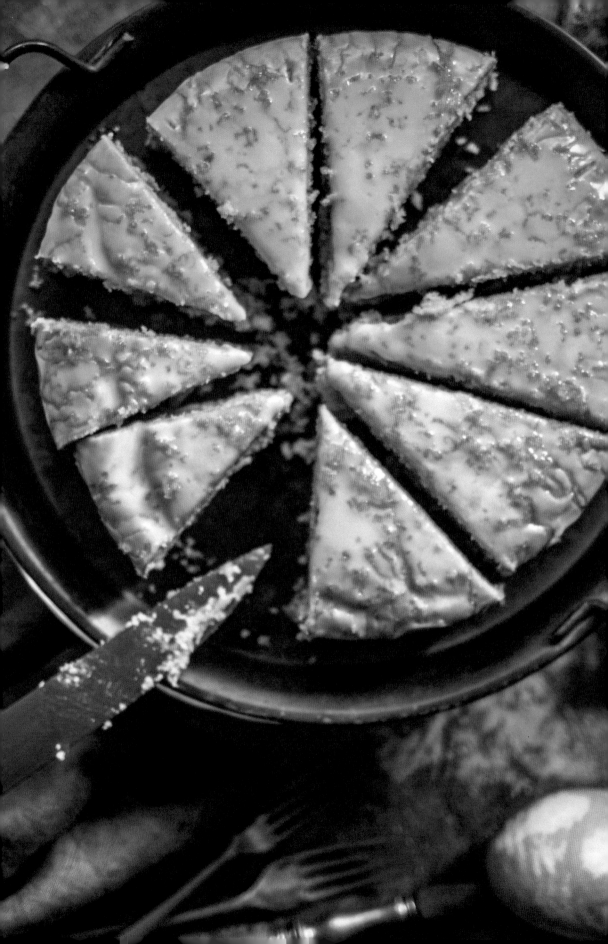

Lemon Drizzle Cake

 10-12 Slices

Ingredients

Cake Mix

- 300g Self Rising Flour
- 1 Tsp Bicarbonate of soda
- 300ml Soya Milk
- 1 Tbsp Apple Cider Vinegar
- 150g Plant margarine at room temperature
- ½ Tsp Salt
- 200g Caster Sugar
- ½ Tsp vanilla essence
- Zest of 2 Lemons

Icing

- 1Cup Icing Sugar
- 1Tbsp lemon juice
- Zest of 1 lemon to decorate

Method

1. Preheat oven at 160 Fan or 180 Conventional ovens.
2. Grease, line and sprinkle with flour, 1x 8 "bake tin.
3. Put the milk and cider vinegar in a jug and set aside.
4. Sift the flour and bicarbonate into a bowl and set aside.
5. In a large mixing bowl, put the margarine, salt, sugar, lemon zest and vanilla and mix with a hand mixer on high speed until the mixture is fluffy and pale in colour, this can take 6-8 minutes.
6. Now you going to mix the rest of the ingredients into the large bowl, alternating the flour and liquid.
7. Start adding some of the flour to the butter mix whilst still mixing the butter mix with the hand mixer. If using a stand mixer leave it on whilst adding the ingredients to it. You start with adding the flour and end with adding the flour. (Flour, liquid, flour, liquid, flour)
8. Once you've added the first bit of flour, whilst mixing, mix till combined then add half of the liquid mixture till combined then add more flour, combine then remainder of the liquid, combine and the remainder flour and combine.. Once this is done use a spatula and go round the sides of the bowl making sure everything is mixed in and well combined. You should have an airy and smooth cake mixture.
9. Pour the cake mixture into the cake tin and bake for 45-55 minutes. Check it after 45 minutes by inserting a wooden skewer in the middle to see if it comes out dry, if not it needs more baking. Sometimes you can see before taking it out of the oven, that it's not ready, the centre will seem like it's still raw, in this case don't remove from the oven and close the oven door quickly so as not to lose too much heat. I would suggest checking it again after 10 minutes before taking it out and doing the skewer test. Once it's done remove from the oven and let it sit in the tin for 10 minutes before transferring it onto a cooling rack.
10. Make the Icing when the cake has cooled down by mixing the frosting ingredients together. It should be a thick pourable consistency. You can add some milk if it's too thick or more icing sugar if too runny.
11. When the cake has cooled down, place it on a cake stand and pour the icing over the cake starting in the centre, using a spatula, spread the icing all over the cake and push it to the edges so it can run down the sides. Sprinkle the cake with lemon zest.

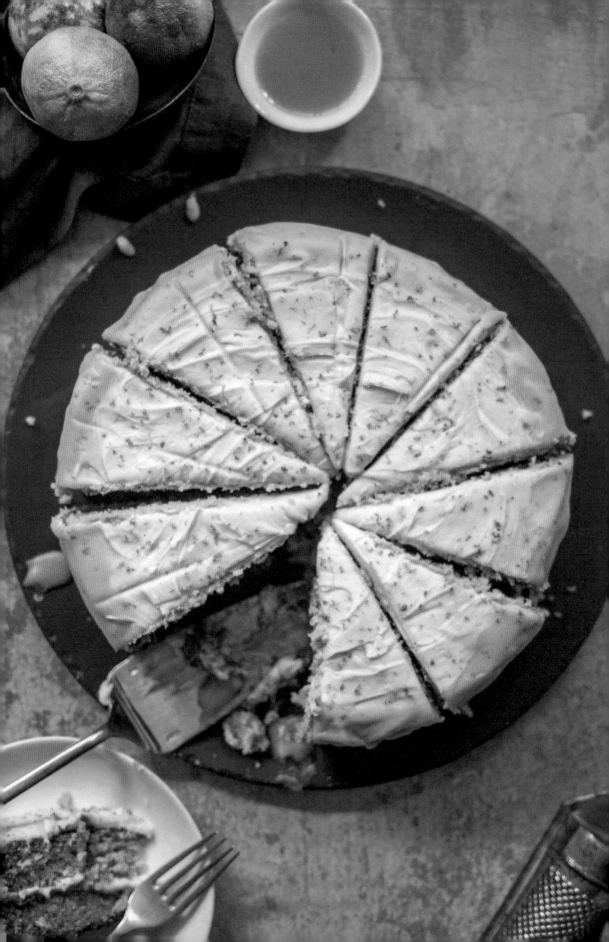

Mango & Lime Cake

 10-12 Slices

Ingredients

- Cake Mix
- 300g Self Rising Flour
- 200ml Soya Milk unsweetened
- 1 Tbsp Apple Cider Vinegar
- 150g Plant margarine at room temperature
- 200g Caster Sugar
- ½ Tsp vanilla essence
- Lime zest of 4 limes (½ mixed in cake ½ to decorate)
- ½ Tsp Salt
- 1 Tsp Bicarbonate of soda
- Juice of 1 lime
- 90-95 ml Mango Pulp
- Frosting
- 450g Icing Sugar
- 45g margarine room temperature
- ½ tsp Vanilla essence
- ¼ Cup mango pulp (More if needed)
- Mango glaze optional
- 1 Cup icing sugar
- 3Tbsp + ½ Tsp Mango Pulp

Method

1. Preheat oven at 160 Fan or 180 Conventional ovens.
2. Grease, line and sprinkle with flour, 1 x 8 "cake tin.
3. Put the milk and cider vinegar in a jug and set aside.
4. In another jug add the lime juice and top up to 100ml with mango pulp (total liquid measures to 100ml
5. Sift the flour and bicarbonate into a bowl and set aside.
6. In a large mixing bowl, put the margarine, salt, sugar, lime zest of 2 limes and vanilla and mix with a hand mixer on high speed until the mixture is fluffy and pale in colour, this can take 6-8 minutes.
7. Now you going to mix the rest of the ingredients into the large bowl, alternating the flour and liquid.
8. Start adding some of the flour to the butter mix whilst still mixing the butter mix with the hand mixer. If using a stand mixer leave it on whilst adding the ingredients to it. You start with adding the flour and end with adding the flour. (Flour, liquid, flour, liquid, flour)
9. Mix the milk mixture and mango mixture together now.
10. Once you've added the first bit of flour, whilst mixing, mix till combined then add half of the liquid mixture till combined then add more flour, combine then remainder of the liquid, combine and the remainder flour and combine.. Once this is done use a spatula and go round the sides of the bowl making sure everything is mixed in and well combined. You should have an airy and smooth cake mixture.
11. Pour the cake mixture into the cake tin and bake for 30-45 minutes. Check it after 30 minutes by inserting a wooden skewer in the middle to see if it comes out dry, if not it needs more baking. Sometimes you can see before taking it out of the oven, that it's not ready, the centre will seem like it's still raw, in this case don't remove from the oven and close the oven door quickly so as not to lose too much heat. I would suggest checking it again after 10 minutes before taking it out and doing the skewer test. Once they done remove from the oven and let it sit in the tin for 10 minutes before transferring it onto a cooling rack.
12. Start to make the frosting, in a large mixing bowl add all the frosting ingredients together keeping ½ of the pulp which you can add bit by bit as mixing. Mix till you have a thick but spreadable consistency. You can add some more pulp or milk if it's too thick or more icing sugar if too runny. Set aside for when the cakes have cooled down
13. To make the glaze, mix the ingredients together, you should have a pouring consistency. You can add more pulp or icing sugar to adjust the thickness. I put mine in a squeeze bottle with a nozzle to make it easier to pour round the edge of the cake.
14. When the cake has cooled down, cut in half and let it cool further. Place the bottom half on a cake stand and frost. Sandwich with the top half, frost the entire cake and sprinkle it with the lime zest.
15. Let the frost set in the fridge for an hour before glazing. Using a squeeze bottle or a jug, pour the glaze round the edge of the cake so that the glaze can drip down the sides.

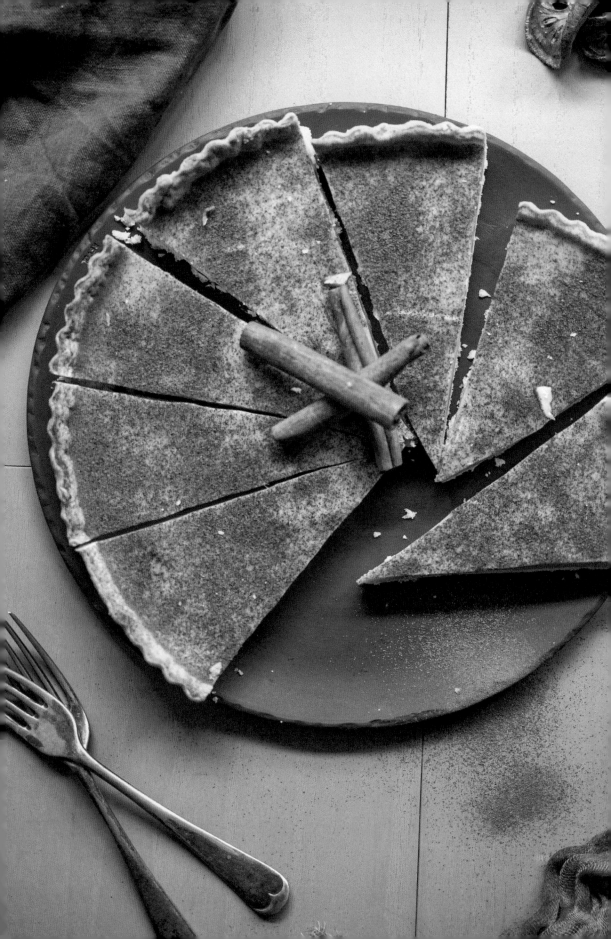

South African Milk Tart

10-12 Slices

Ingredients

- 1x 375g Short crust pastry room temperature
- 1x Can 200g Plant condensed milk
- 800ml Soya milk unsweetened
- 3 Tbsp Custard Powder
- 3 Tbsp + 1 Tsp Corn Flour
- 2 Tbsp Sugar
- Cinnamon to sprinkle

Method

1. Preheat the oven to 180 fan or 200 conventional ovens.

2. Place the puff pastry into a 30cm tart baking pan. The pastry will not be wide enough but will be longer than needed and hang over on one side, cut that off and add it to the width where needed. Simply cut it off and stick it onto the area that's needed by pressing the pastry to stick together.

3. Using a fork, make holes in the pastry and bake for 15-20 min or until lightly golden brown.

4. Once baked, set it aside to cool.

5. In a large measuring jug, add the condensed milk and top up with milk up to 1lt in total and mix well.

6. Take some of the milk from the jug and pour it into a cup.

7. Mix the custard and cornflower into the cup of milk and stir it making sure there are no lumps and its all turned to liquid

8. In a large pan on a high heat, pour the milk from the jug into the pan add the sugar and stir. Bring to the boil. Whilst you waiting for the milk to boil, keep stirring the milk in the cup with the custard and corn flour.

9. When the milk starts to boil, simmer the heat and immediately add the cup of custard milk into the pan and stir continuously for 5 minutes. It will start to thicken, keep an eye on it as it could burn if you don't keep stirring it. If it's too hot simmer the heat further.

10. Pour the custard mix onto the pastry in the tart pan.

11. Sprinkle the cinnamon on whilst the custard is still hot.

12. Leave it to cool and then place it in the fridge to set for at least 2 hours.

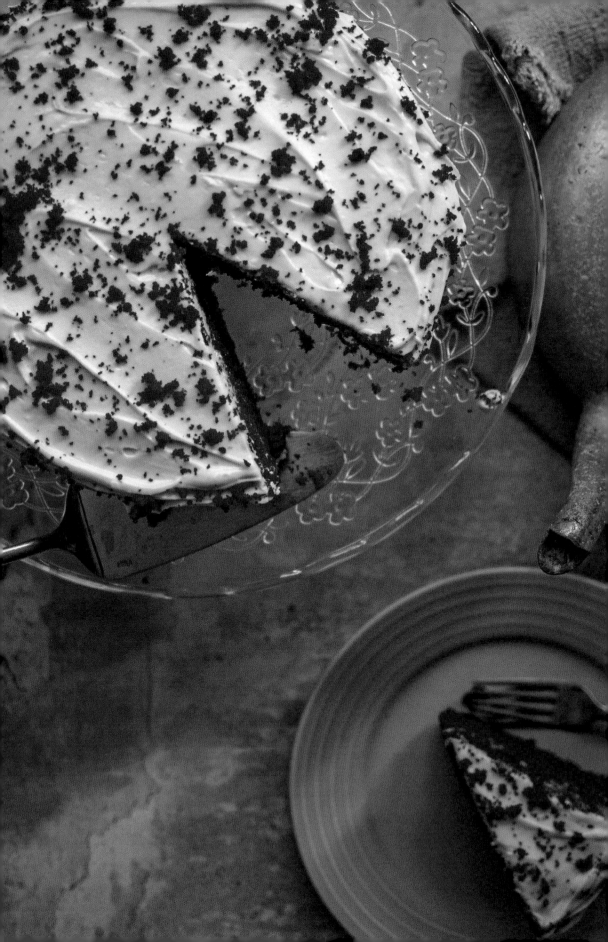

Red Velvet Cake

 10-12 Slices

Ingredients

Cake Mix

- 300g Self Rising Flour
- 1 Tsp Bicarbonate of soda
- 1 Tbsp Cacao powder
- 300ml Soya Milk
- 1 Tbsp Apple Cider Vinegar
- 150g Plant margarine at room temperature
- ½ Tsp Salt
- 200g Caster Sugar
- ½ Tsp vanilla essence
- 2 – 2 & ½ Tsp Red Dye paste (If your dye is a liquid, then you should reduce the milk in the same quantity as the amount of dye you using)

Frosting

- 450g Icing Sugar
- 45g Margarine
- Juice of 1 Lemon
- 1 Tsp Vanilla essence
- Milk if needed

Method

1. Preheat oven at 160 Fan or 180 Conventional ovens.
2. Grease, line and sprinkle with flour, 1 x 8 "bake tin.
3. Put the milk and cider vinegar in a jug and set aside.
4. Sift the flour, cacao and bicarbonate into a bowl, mix with a whisk & set aside.
5. In a large mixing bowl, put the margarine, salt, sugar and vanilla and mix with a hand mixer on high speed until the mixture is fluffy and pale in colour, this can take 6-8 minutes.
6. Now you going to mix the rest of the ingredients into the large bowl, alternating the flour and liquid.
7. Start adding some of the flour to the butter mix whilst still mixing the butter mix with the hand mixer. If using a stand mixer leave it on whilst adding the ingredients to it. You start with adding the flour and end with adding the flour. (Flour, liquid, flour, liquid, flour)
8. Once you've added the first bit of flour, whilst mixing, mix till combined then add half of the liquid mixture till combined then add more flour, combine then remainder of the liquid, combine and the remainder flour and combine.. Now add the dye and mix well, your cake mix should be a dark pink / red to achieve a nice red when baked. I find that a vegan extra red paste works best. Once this is done use a spatula and go round the sides of the bowl making sure everything is mixed in and well combined. You should have an airy and smooth cake mixture.
9. Pour the cake mixture into the cake tin and bake for 35-45 minutes some ovens may take longer. Check by inserting a wooden skewer in the middle to see if it comes out dry, if not it needs more baking. Sometimes you can see before taking it out of the oven, that it's not ready, the centre will seem like it's still raw, in this case don't remove from the oven and close the oven door quickly so as not to lose too much heat. I would suggest checking it again after 10 minutes before taking it out and doing the skewer test. Once it's done remove from the oven and let it sit in the tin for 10 minutes before transferring it onto a cooling rack.
10. When the cake has cooled down, cut the cake in half so you can add frosting in the middle of the cake, it will need to cool further once cut.
11. Mix the frosting ingredients together using a hand mixer till you have a thick but spreadable frosting. If it's too thick, add a tsp of milk at a time until you get the correct consistency.
12. When the cake has cooled down, rub the sponge a little to get some crumbs from it so you can sprinkle them on top of the cake once it's frosted. Place the bottom half on a cake stand and use a cake spatula to frost it. Then sandwich the top to the bottom and frost the entire cake. Sprinkle with the crumbs. Let it set in the fridge for an hour before cutting.

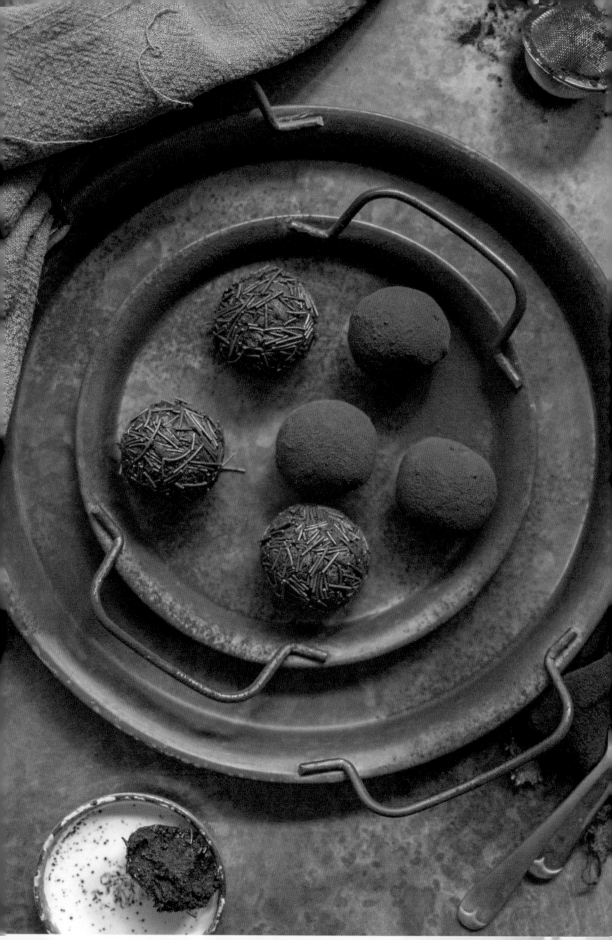

Rum & Raisin Chocolate balls

 Makes 8-12

Ingredients

Cake (can make the day before)

- 250g Self Rising Flour
- 50g Cacao Powder
- 1 Tsp Bicarbonate of soda
- 300ml Soya Milk
- 1 Tbsp Apple Cider Vinegar
- 150g Plant margarine at room temperature
- ½ Tsp Salt
- 200g Caster Sugar
- ½ Tsp vanilla essence

Ingredients to add to the chocolate cake to make the balls

- ¼ Cup chopped raisins
- ¼ Cup Dark Rum
- ¼ Cup + 1Tbsp Condensed Milk
- Chocolate sprinkles or cacao powder to coat

Method

Make the chocolate cake first. You need 340g of chocolate cake for the recipe. This cake recipe makes 850g. You could freeze the extra cake to use another time or you could double up on the balls ingredients to use up the cake.

1. Preheat oven at 160 Fan or 180 Conventional ovens.
2. Grease, line and sprinkle with flour, 1x 8 "bake tin.
3. Put the milk and cider vinegar in a jug and set aside.
4. Sift the flour, cacao and bicarbonate into a bowl and set aside.
5. In a large mixing bowl, put the margarine, salt, sugar and vanilla and mix with a hand mixer on high speed until the mixture is fluffy and pale in colour, this can take 6-8 minutes.
6. Now you going to mix the rest of the ingredients into the large bowl, alternating the flour and liquid.
7. Start adding some of the flour to the butter mix whilst still mixing the butter mix with the hand mixer. If using a stand mixer leave it on whilst adding the ingredients to it. You start with adding the flour and end with adding the flour. (Flour, liquid, flour, liquid, flour)
8. Once you've added the first bit of flour, whilst mixing, mix till combined then add half of the liquid mixture till combined then add more flour, combine then remainder of the liquid, combine and the remainder flour and combine.. Once this is done use a spatula and go round the sides of the bowl making sure everything is mixed in and well combined. You should have an airy and smooth cake mixture.
9. Pour the cake mixture into the cake tin and bake for 45-55 minutes. Check it after 45 minutes by inserting a wooden skewer in the middle to see if it comes out dry, if not it needs more baking. Sometimes you can see before taking it out of the oven, that it's not ready, the centre will seem like it's still raw, in this case don't remove from the oven and close the oven door quickly so as not to lose too much heat. I would suggest checking it again after 10 minutes before taking it out and doing the skewer test. Once it's done remove from the oven and let it sit in the tin for 10 minutes before transferring it onto a cooling rack.
10. When you cake has completely cooled down, break it up into crumbs and place 340g in a mixing bowl
11. In a small pan on a med-high heat, add the raisins and 1 & ½ Tbsp of rum, stir for about 5 minutes or until the raisins have softened or absorbed all the rum. Set aside to cool.
12. Add the remainder of the ingredients including the cooled down raisins into the bowl with the cake and mix it all together.
13. On a side plate add the chocolate sprinkles or cacao powder to roll the balls in
14. Using your hands, make balls out of the mixture and then roll them over the sprinkles or cacao making sure the balls are fully coated
15. Once coated, put them in the fridge, they should last 5 days and they can also be frozen.

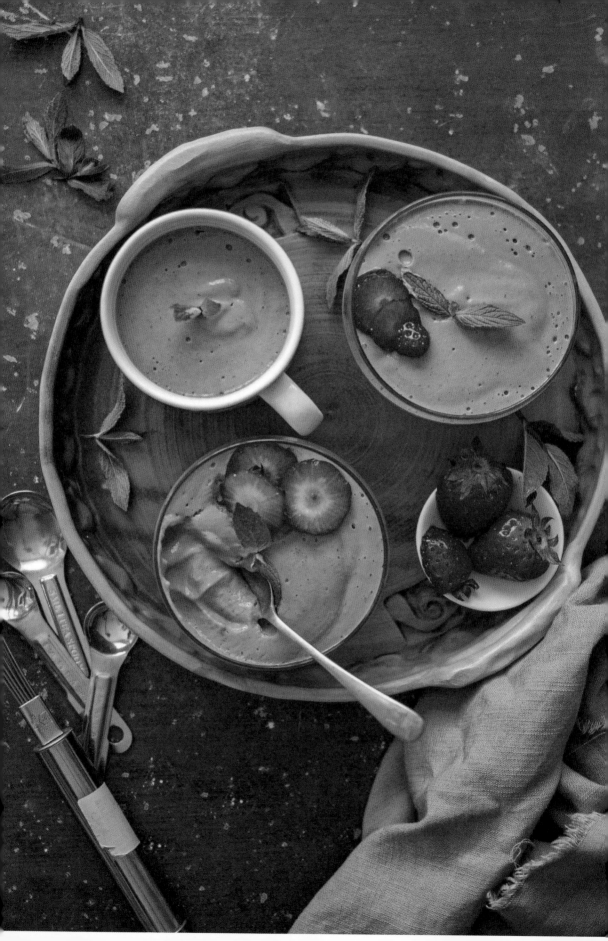

Strawberry & Mint Mousse

Makes 2-4

Ingredients

- 110g Fresh strawberries, extra for garnish
- 4-6 leaves fresh mint, plus more for garnish
- 349g silken tofu
- 1/3 cup Caster sugar
- Pink food colouring optional
- Maple Syrup optional

Method

1. Mix all the ingredients in a food processor or blender (blender will give it more silky texture) Blend till everything is well combined and smooth.

2. Pour into teacups, ramekins or mousse bowls and let them set overnight in the fridge. If using maple syrup, pour it over the mousse before serving and garnish with some fresh strawberries and mint.

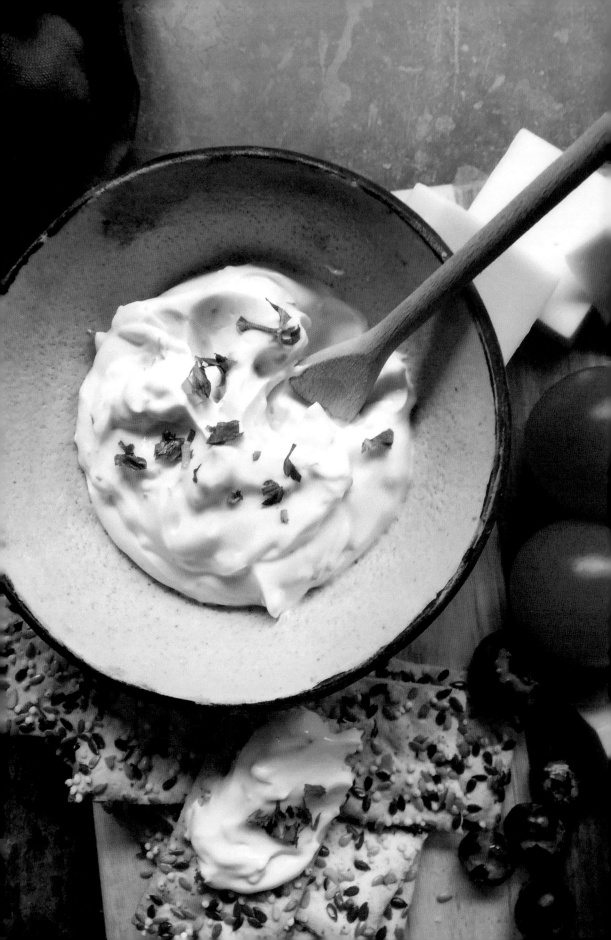

Dips
or
Sauces

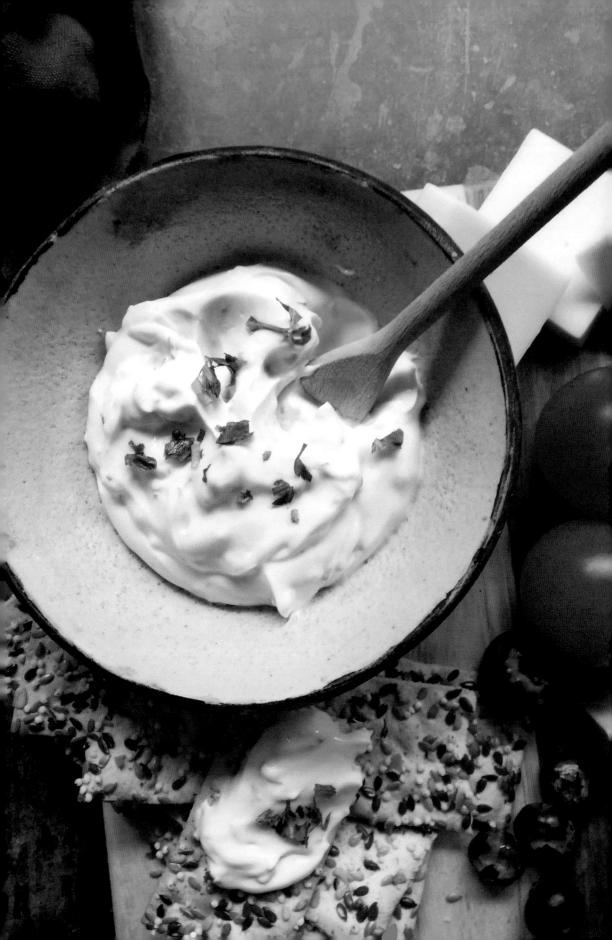

Soya Cream Cheese

Serves 2-4 or more if using the tofu

Ingredients

- 1 Pot 340g Soya yogurt
- Some herbs of your choice (I used a palm full of chives)
- 2-3 Tbsp Nutritional Yeast (optional, has a nutty and cheesy flavour)
- Salt & Pepper to taste
- ½-1 Tsp vinegar (any)
- 1 Box 349g Silken Tofu (optional) I used to thicken the cheese, you could also use firm tofu)

Method

1. This recipe needs to start the day before to give the yogurt time to drain all the liquid. Use a tea towel instead of muslin as the yogurt will go straight through the muslin. You need a large jar with a lid so you have space for the water to drain from the yogurt without touching the yogurt once drained. Place the towel in the jar and pour the yogurt into the cloth. If you don't have a lid to hold the cloth in place, fasten with elastic or string at the top to prevent it from moving downwards. It needs to be in place and have free space for the liquid at the bottom. Place the lid on and put it into the fridge overnight. If your jar doesn't have a lid, cover it up with another tea towel.

2. Take the yogurt out of the fridge after an overnight drain, you will see it has thickened and the drained water at the bottom of the jar. To make this without the tofu, simply put the thickened yogurt and remaining ingredients into a bowl and mix well.

3. If you want it to be thicker, use the tofu. Using a hand blender or food processor, blend the tofu till smooth. Transfer to a bowl and add the remainder ingredients and mix well.

4. You can store it in the fridge in an airtight container for 4 days. When using the tofu, if you let it set overnight once it's all mixed together, it will thicken and set a bit more. You could also use a different plant yogurt that's thicker than soya and follow the steps to make the cream cheese and the results will be a thicker more set cream cheese.

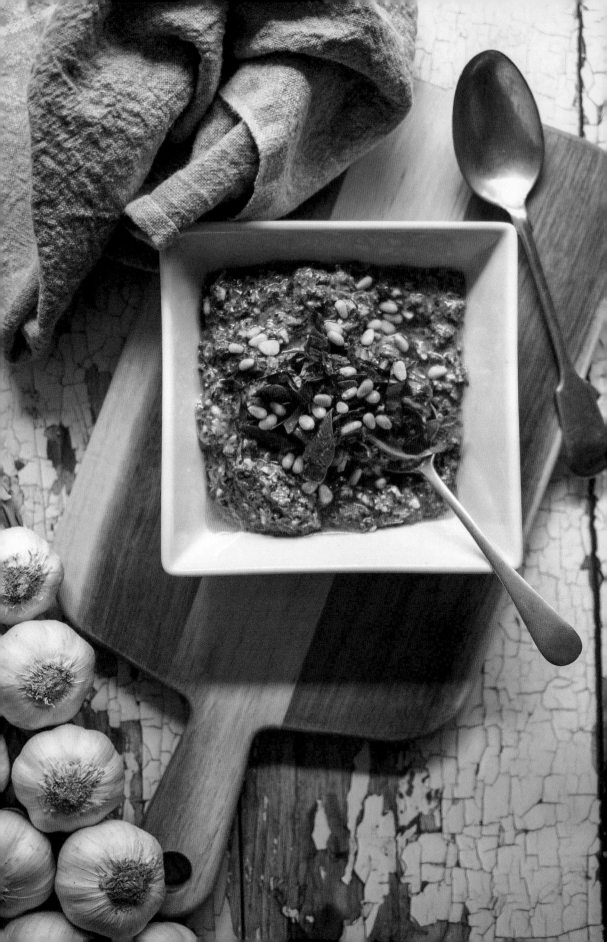

Kale & Spinach Pesto

Serves 4 for pasta dish recipe or 6-8 for bagels recipe in this book

This is a very fresh and nutritious pesto. I absolutely love it and eat it raw. You can eat it raw or heat it up. It has more nutritional value raw as when you heat it, it loses some nutrients but it's still good for you either way.

Ingredients

- 180g chopped kale
- 125g baby leaf spinach
- ½ cup mixed chopped nuts
- Handful of pine nuts
- 4 large garlic cloves
- 1 cup Olive Oil
- ½ cup vegetable Oil
- 4 Tbsp Nutritional Yeast (Optional)
- Juice of 1 large Lemon
- Salt and pepper to taste

Method

1. Firstly put nuts, not the pine nuts into a food processor and blitz till roughly chopped for a nice texture & leave them in the processor.

2. Then add the kale and blitz again, add some of the olive oil here to allow it to mix well and until it's a nice fine texture.

3. Now add the rest of the ingredients except the pine nuts and hold back the ½ cup of sunflower oil which you can add right at the end if needed.

4. Mix well in the processor to your desired texture, taste and season with salt & pepper, add the pine nuts and use the pulse on the processor for a final mix.

TIP:

Store in an airtight container in the fridge for 4-5 days. If you don't like too much oil in your pesto, you can put less oil and top up with water. This also freezes well for 3 months and when you need it, you can simply take it out the freezer and let it defrost, it will be as fresh as when you made it.

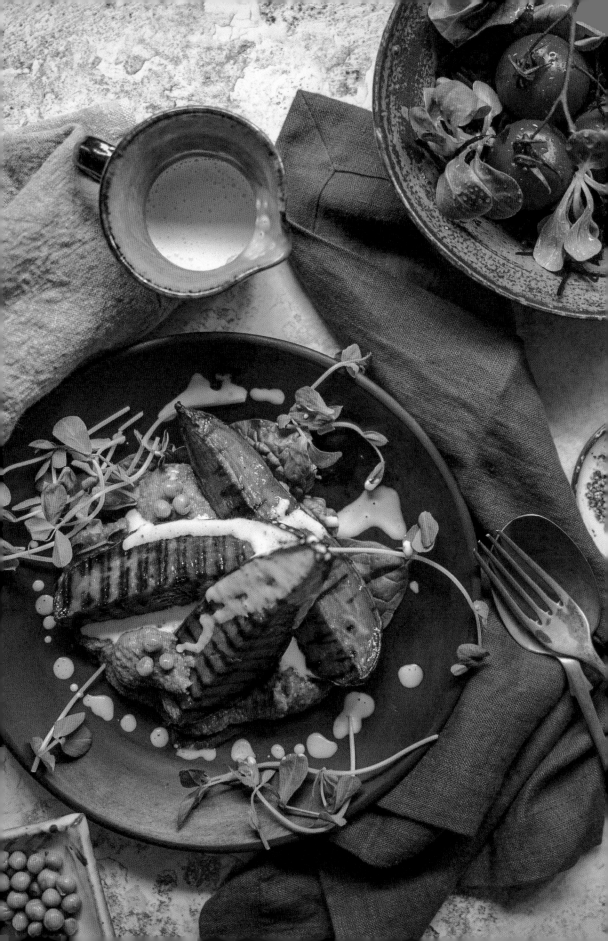

Light Meals

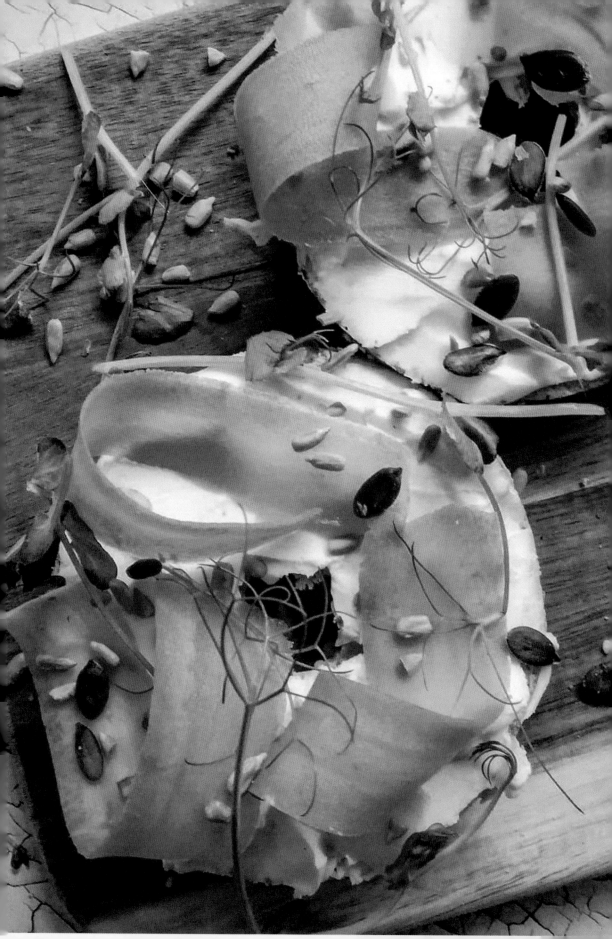

Cream Cheese Bagels with Carrot or Pesto

Serves 2

Ingredients

- 2 bagels
- Shop bought cream cheese or my recipe in this book
- Shop bought pesto or my recipe in this book
- 1 carrot peeled length ways
- Handful of pea shoots or other micro greens
- Handful of mixed seeds

Method

1. Cut and toast bagels. Let them cool a bit before spreading the cream cheese so it doesn't melt. You can serve them open as in the picture or closed if packing them for lunch. Spread the cheese on both halves. Using a potato peeler, peel the carrot length ways to get nice long thin slices, curl them up and place on top of the cheese. Sprinkle the micro greens then seeds and serve. Do the same for the pesto, start with the cheese then spread the pesto, seeds and micro greens.

2. If using my pesto recipe, half the recipe as it makes a lot. You can also freeze the pesto in little posts and take it out the day before to defrost so you don't have wastage.

3. If you going to use my cheese recipe remember to do it a day before hand so it has time to thicken and set.

4. There are a lot of great plant based cream cheeses available to buy if you don't have the time to do the prep beforehand and you need a quick lunch x

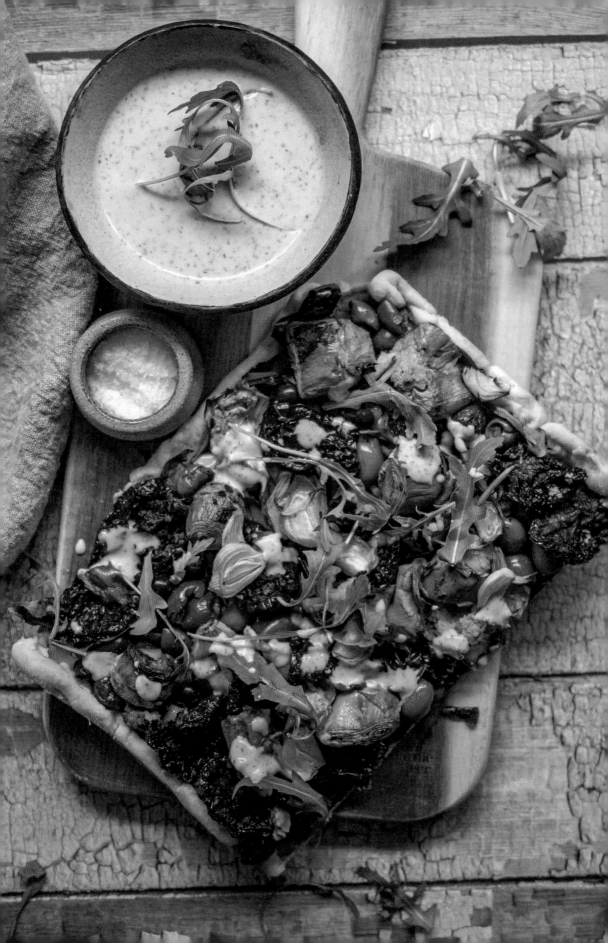

Mediterranean Tart with Yogurt Drizzle

Serves 4-6

Ingredients

- 1 Packet 375g puff pastry at room temperature
- 150g ready cooked artichokes from a jar drained & roughly chopped
- 4 Shallots sliced
- 270g mixed pitted olives roughly chopped
- 300g Sun dried tomatoes roughly chopped
- 150g baby leaf spinach
- Rocket Leaves for garnish.
- Yogurt Drizzle
- 1 cup soy yogurt
- 50g of mixed baby spinach & rocket leaves
- 1Tsp olive oil
- I Tsp lemon juice
- Salt & pepper to taste

Method

1. Preheat oven to 180 fan / 200 conventional ovens. Lightly grease a 14" baking try.

2. Place the puff pastry on the baking tray and make holes using a fork into the pastry, bake for 15 minutes or till light golden in colour.

3. Remove from the oven and start to fill, I started with a layer of spinach leaves first and then added the remainder of the ingredients on top of that. Put it back in the oven for a further 15-20 minutes.

4. Using a hand blender or a food processor, mix the yogurt with the leaves until smooth. Then add the lemon, oil, salt and pepper to taste. Drizzle over the tart once it's done.

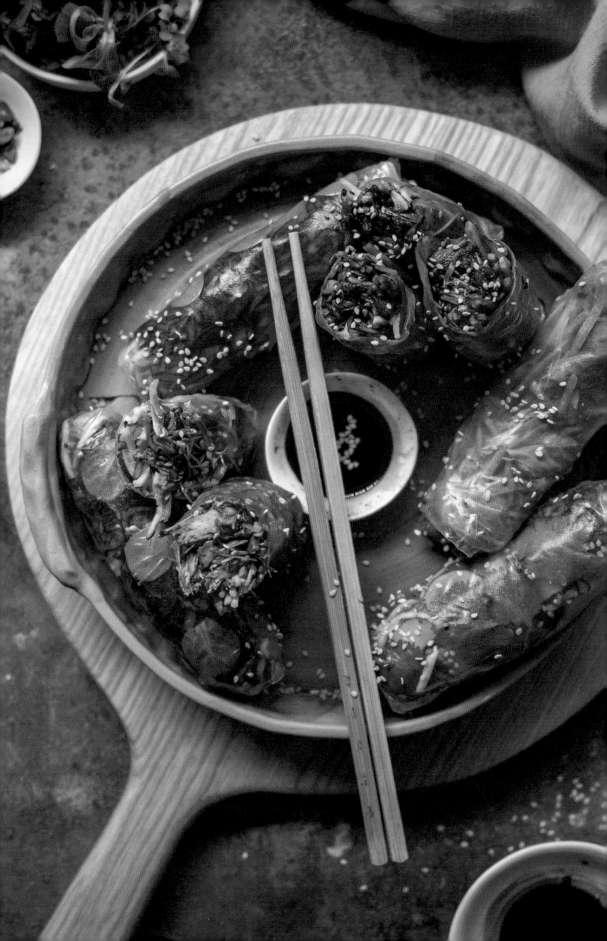

Jackfruit Rice Paper Wraps / Spring Rolls

Makes 5 Med – Large Rolls

Ingredients

- For the Jackfruit
- 2 Tbsp Bbq sauce
- 1 Tsp Dark Soya Sauce
- ½ Tsp Vegetable oil
- 400g (1 Tin) drained Young Jackfruit
- For The rice paper wraps
- A dinner plate filled with cold water to soak the rice paper.
- 1 carrot finely grated / shredded
- 1 courgette finely grated / shredded
- Red cabbage finely sliced/ shredded (as much as you like)
- ½ bunch of parsley, using the full leaves
- 4 Radishes finely sliced
- Cress sprouts, as much as you like for filling and garnishing
- Handful of pumpkin, sesame and sunflower seeds
- Mixed chopped nuts optional
- Dark Soya sauce to serve

Method

1. Preparation is important for this dish. Firstly make the jackfruit, let it cool and cut up all your ingredients. They should be finely grated or chopped so they don't rip the paper. Once the rice paper has softened, sharp or chunky ingredients can rip the paper whilst wrapping them.

2. Drain the jackfruit and shred it with your hands, if there are any harder bits finely chop them. On a med to high heat, mix all the jackfruit ingredients well and cook for 2 to 3 minutes, set aside to cool down.

3. Have all your ingredients ready and laid out in front of you before starting. When this is done you can start to fill the wraps. Take a rice paper wrap and dip it into the water, making sure you wet the whole thing. You don't have to wait for it to soften in the water as it will soften whilst you fill it with ingredients. I wet it and remove it from the water straight away. Place the wet paper on a flat surface and start filling. Leave a 2cm space on the paper that's closest to you so you can roll it over when the ingredients are on and 1 cm spaces on the sides so you can fold the sides in. I start with leaves and place them upside down so they are visible when rolled. Then I add the cabbage, jackfruit carrots, courgettes, seeds/nuts, radish and lastly the sprouts so they visible as well. You can play around with this and use different leaves or ingredients and when you get the hang of it, you can really make them look amazing once rolled up.

4. To wrap them, start with the top closest to you, gently pull it over the filling (don't overfill them) and try to tuck it under, then fold the sides in and keep rolling till the end. If you've never done it before, it could be a bit tricky at first but you will soon get the hang of it after trying to make a few. Serve with dark soya sauce to dip the wraps into.

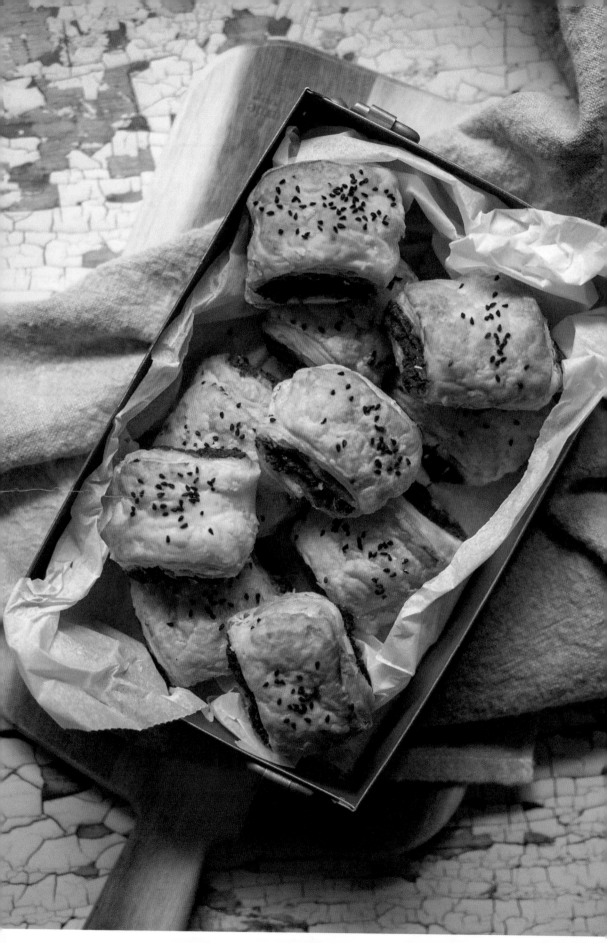

Mushroom & Chestnut Mini Sausage Rolls

Makes 16

Ingredients

- 1 Pack 375g Puff Pastry room temperature
- 2 Portobello Mushrooms roughly chopped
- 2 chestnut mushrooms roughly chopped
- 90g whole cooked chestnuts roughly chopped
- 120g Firm tofu (pressed) roughly chopped
- ½ Red onion roughly chopped
- 1 sprig of rosemary
- 1 Garlic Clove roughly chopped
- 1 tsp English Mustard
- Salt & pepper to taste
- 1 Tsp Olive Oil
- ½ Tsp Smoked Paprika
- Soya Milk to brush pastry
- Nigella or poppy seeds to sprinkle
- Breadcrumbs if needed

Method

1. In a food processor, put all the ingredients except the oil, salt, pepper and breadcrumbs. Mix till you have a fine / pate texture. In a pan heat the oil on a med-high heat and add mixture to the pan, stir continuously for 3 minutes or until there is no liquid left in the mixture. Remove from the heat to cool, taste and season. If your mixture is not firm enough to hold together add some breadcrumbs and mix well. Start with a table spoon at a time.

2. On a floured surface, roll out your pastry and cut it in half lengthways. Place some of the mixture in the centre of one of the halves, leaving about a 1cm gap at both ends to be able to seal it closed. Pull one side of the pastry over the filling to form the roll shape. Turn the pastry as you roll and when you get to the end, brush some milk on the pastry to glue it together. Now turn the roll round so that the fold is underneath. When you bake it the fold also needs to be underneath so it doesn't come undone.

3. Using a sharp knife, start to cut the roll into small rolls. Start by cutting in half, then half the half and so on. One half will give you 6- 8 mini rolls. Repeat these steps with the remaining half of the pastry. Now place all the rolls on a greased baking pan, brush with milk and sprinkle with the seeds. Place the tray in the fridge for 10- 20 minutes to firm up. Preheat the oven to 200 fan or 220 conventional ovens. Bake for 25-30 minutes or until golden brown.

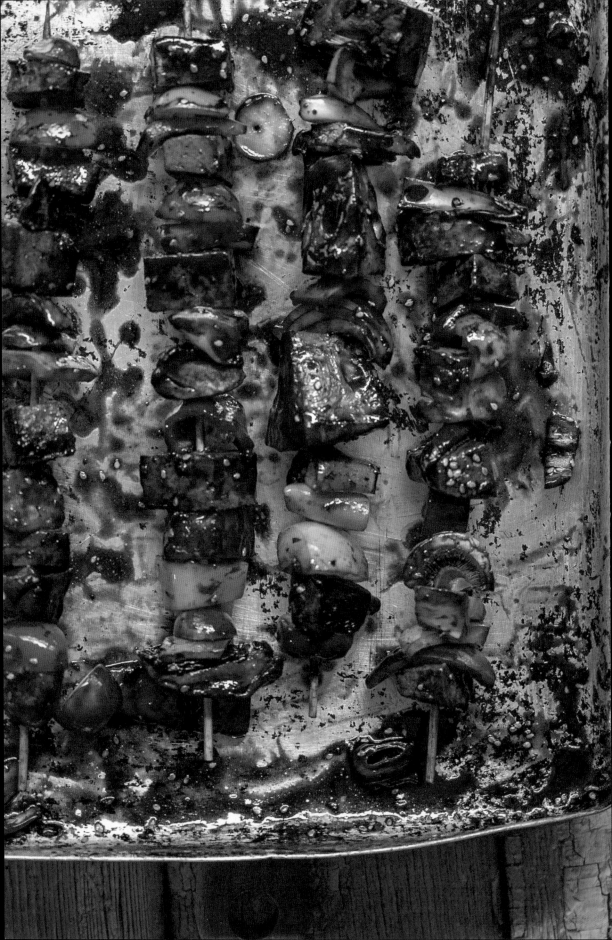

Sweet & Sour Skewers with (Tofu or Jackfruit)

Makes 12 – 18

Ingredients

For the skewer

- 1 packet button mushrooms whole / cut in half
- 1 Red, 1 Green & 1 Yellow bell pepper cut in chunks
- 2-3 red or green fresh chillies optional cut in chunks
- ½ Pineapple cut in chunks
- 300g firm tofu cut in cubes or 400g tin Jackfruit drained and used whole
- 2 Red onions cut in chunks
- 8-12 radishes halved
- 8-12 cherry tomatoes whole or cut in half

For the marinade

- 4 Tbsp Bbq Sauce
- 3 Tbsp dark Soy sauce
- 2-3 Tbsp Vegetable Oil
- Palm full of sesame seeds optional

Method

1. Chop up all your ingredients to a similar size 3-4cm. If you cut them too small they will fall off the skewer. Place all your chopped ingredients in a row in front of you to make it easier when putting all the ingredients together onto the skewers.

2. Mix your marinade ingredients into a bowl and place the tofu or jackfruit into the marinade and make sure it's all covered and coated well. You can make a double portion of marinade to have extra to brush over the skewers before and after cooking.

3. I started with the radish as its firm and won't slip off the skewer. Start filling your skewers and you can end with radish or onions, something to keep them in place. Once you've done all the skewers, brush them over with some marinade making sure you coat all the ingredients.

4. You can cook these in several ways, on a Bbq or on a tray in the oven 180-200 fan for 15-20 minutes or on a grill or skillet on the hob on a med – high heat turning every 2-5 minutes for around 10-15 minutes. Once they done, you can brush over some more marinade before serving.

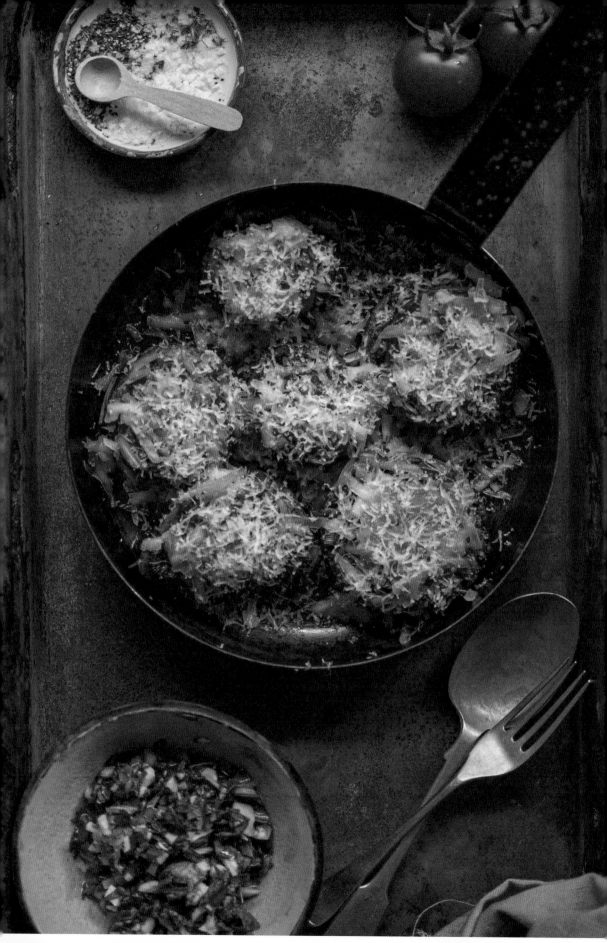

Stuffed Garlic Mushrooms

Serves 2-4

Ingredients

- 4 Portobello mushrooms (stalks removed and keep)
- 2 Tomatoes sliced
- Parsley to garnish finely chopped
- 6 Garlic cloves finely chopped
- 100g baby spinach leaves finely chopped
- Mushroom stalks finely chopped
- 2 Spring onions finely chopped
- Juice of ½ a lemon
- 1 sprig of thyme optional/ 1 tsp
- 1 Tbsp Olive Oil
- Salt & pepper t taste
- 1 cup grated cheese. I used mozzarella and cheddar mixed

Method

1. Preheat Oven 180 fan or 200 conventional ovens.

2. Remove the stalks from the mushrooms and set aside, finely chop the stalks with the rest of the ingredients except the tomatoes and put into a mixing bowl. Add the lemon juice, oil and thyme, mix well, taste and season.

3. Place the mushrooms on a baking tray and fill them with the mixture. Slice the tomatoes and place a full round slice on top of the filling. You may have some filling leftover which you can serve raw with the mushrooms once they done.

4. Place the mushrooms in the oven for 20-25 min. After 20 minutes, take the mushrooms out and top with cheese and bake for a further 5 minutes. Serve with the leftover mix or a nice salad and garnish with parsley before serving.

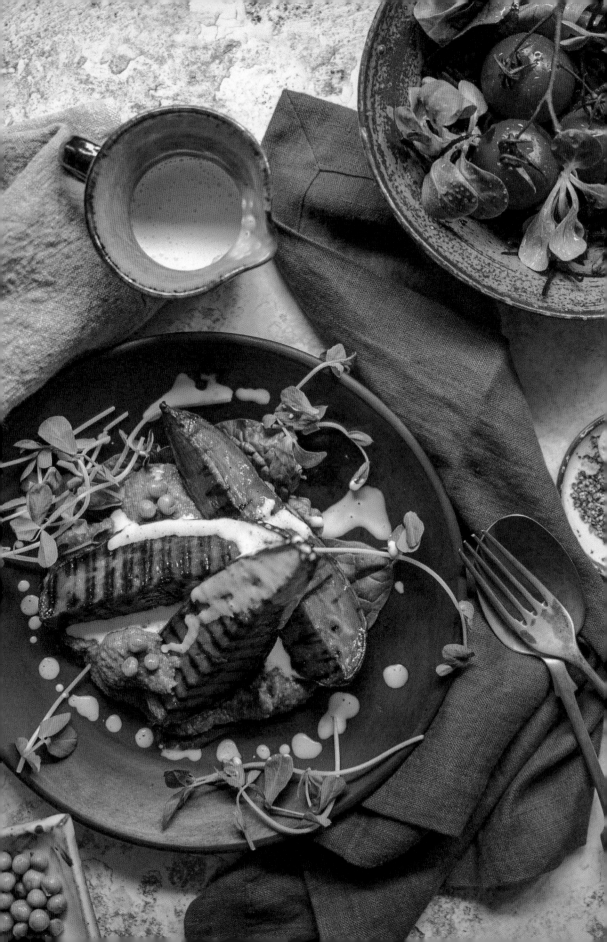

Baked Sweet Potato with Spinach and Pea Mint Puree

 Serves 2

Ingredients

- 2 med- large sweet potatoes, skins left on & cut into ¼ wedges
- 150-200g baby spinach leaves
- ½ cup soya yogurt
- Pea shoots/ micro greens to garnish
- 1 tbsp Olive oil

Mint Pure

- 300g frozen peas defrosted
- 4 Sprigs of fresh mint
- 1 Tsp Olive oil
- Salt and pepper to taste

Method

1. Preheat oven 200 fan or 220 conventional ovens. Rinse the potatoes and cut them lengthways, first in half then the halves in half so you have 4 wedges per potato. Leave the potato skins on. You can remove them after baking if you don't like eating the skins. Rub them with olive oil and place them on a baking tray and bake for 20-30 minutes. If you want to get the grill lines onto the potatoes, you can do so after they've baked by placing them on a grill plate or pan and grill for a minute or 2 until the grill lines are visible.

2. To make the pea pure, bring a cup of water to the boil on a high heat. Add the defrosted peas and boil for 2 minutes. Don't boil for longer as they will lose their vibrant green colour. Drain the water and add the mint and oil to the drained peas. Using a hand blender or food processor, blend the peas till smooth, taste and season. Get this ready 5 minutes before your potatoes are done.

3. For the spinach leaves, in a pan put half a cup of water and bring to the boil, add the spinach to the pan and cook for a minute or so and drain the water. Do this after you've done the pea pure.

4. To plate up, start by putting the pure on the plate and then spinach on top of that. Now place your potatoes on top of the spinach at an angle so they stand up on the plate. Drizzle with yogurt and garnish with seeds and micro greens. You can serve this dish with a mixed leaf salad.

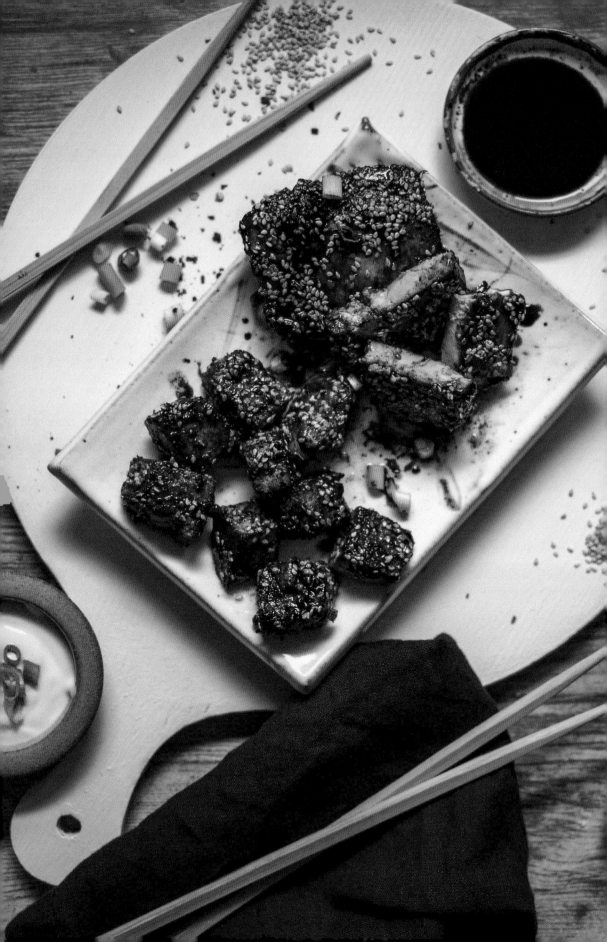

Pan Fried Tofu with Sesame Seeds

Serves 2

I enjoy tofu and have used it in many ways. It's a great ingredient and very nutritious. With this recipe, you can use this in a burger, a salad, just as a snack, serve with rice, in a wrap or have it as a tofu steak.

Ingredients

- 280g Firm Plain/ Smoked Tofu Sliced or cubed
- 2 Tbsp sesame seeds (add as much as you like)
- 3 Tbsp Miso Paste
- 1 Tbsp water
- 1-3 Tbsp Vegetable oil
- 1 Tbsp Dark Soy Sauce plus more for serving
- 2 Tbsp Bbq Sauce
- Soya Yogurt for dipping or drizzling (Optional)
- 1 Spring Onion finely chopped to garnish

Method

1. Cut the tofu into cubes or 1cm steaks. In a bowl mix the miso with water to make a runny but thick enough paste to coat the tofu. To the paste add 1 Tbsp oil, soy sauce and bbq sauce. Mix well.

2. Place the tofu into the paste and coat well on all sides. Leave it in the paste till you start frying. Put a Tbsp of oil In a non- stick pan, on med-high heat and place the tofu into the pan, cooking both sides for about 3 minutes each side.

3. Now coat the tofu in the pan with the seeds and cook for a minute, turn over and coat with seeds on the other side and cook for another minute for the seeds to stick to the tofu.

4. Serve with dark soy sauce, soy yogurt and sprinkle with spring onion

Tip:

If tofu is new to you, I suggest leaving it to marinade in the paste for a few hours or overnight so it can absorb the flavours more. You could also make extra paste to dip the tofu in after cooking. Tofu can be eaten raw or cooked so it doesn't really matter if you cook it for a minute or for 5. I cook it longer when I'm in a char grilled mood and burn it a bit and other times I just cook it for a minute.

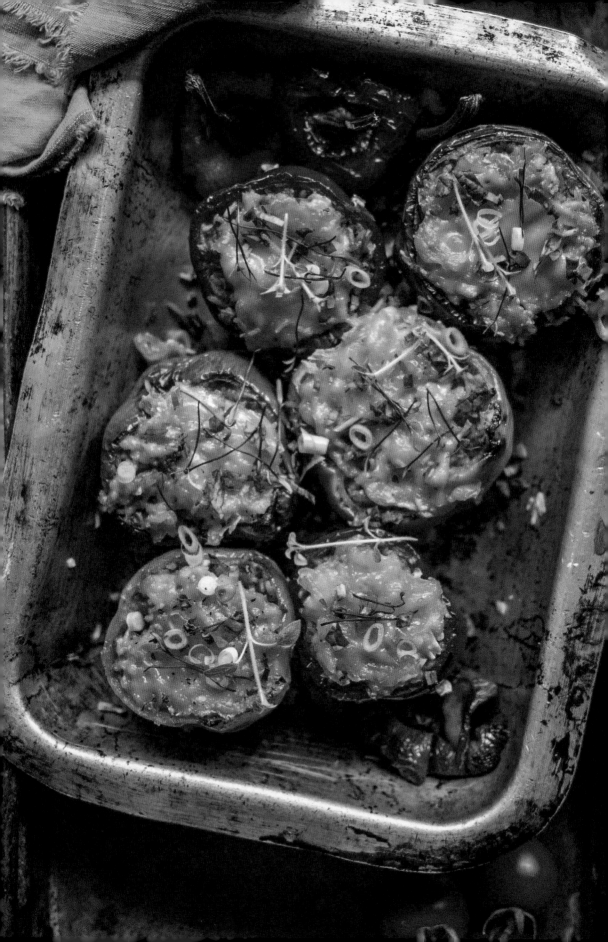

Main Meals

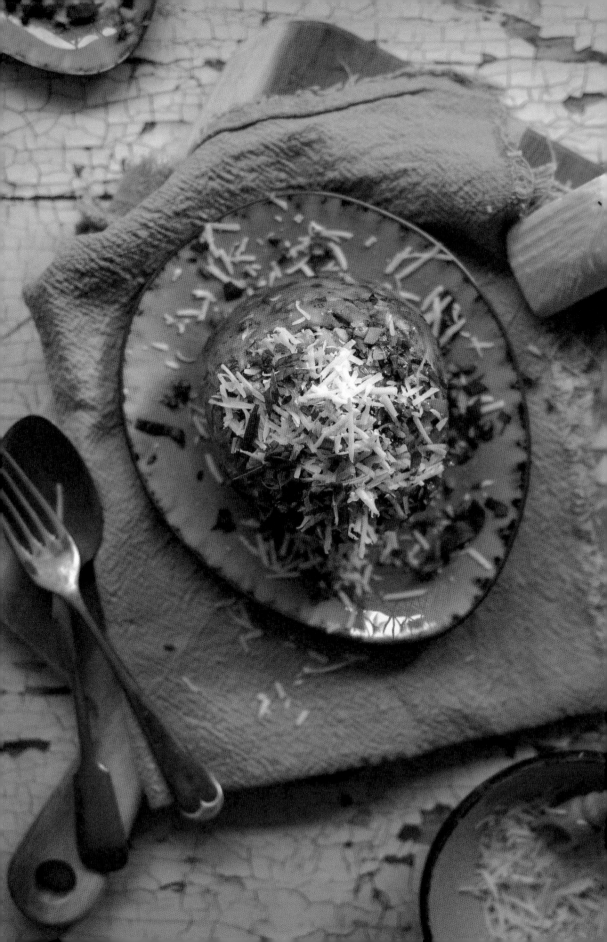

Stuffed Celeriac

Serves 1

Ingredients

- 1 Med Size Celeriac, scrubbed clean and skin left on
- 1 x Sprig Rosemary
- 2 Garlic Cloves roughly chopped
- 2 Tbsp Olive oil

Stuffing

- 1 Portobello Mushroom finely chopped
- Handful Baby leaf Spinach Finely Chopped
- 1 Spring Onion Finely Chopped
- 50-70g Mozzarella or preferred cheese
- Salt & pepper to taste

Method

1. Preheat oven to 160 fan or 180 conventional ovens. Rub the celeriac, with oil, rosemary and garlic. Wrap it in foil, root side down and seal well so the heat doesn't escape from the foil.

2. Place on a baking tray and leave in the oven for 2 hours. Remove from the oven and let it cool down before cutting the top off and removing the centre with a sharp knife and spoon to scoop it out.

3. If you accidently cut the celeriac whilst removing the inside, simply wrap it in foil to hold its shape.

4. Cut up the removed celeriac and mix with all the stuffing ingredients, keep some cheese aside to sprinkle on top of the stuffing. Stuff the celeriac and put it back in the oven for a further 15-25 minutes. .

5. The skin of a celeriac is edible. Serve this with a salad or steamed vegetables.

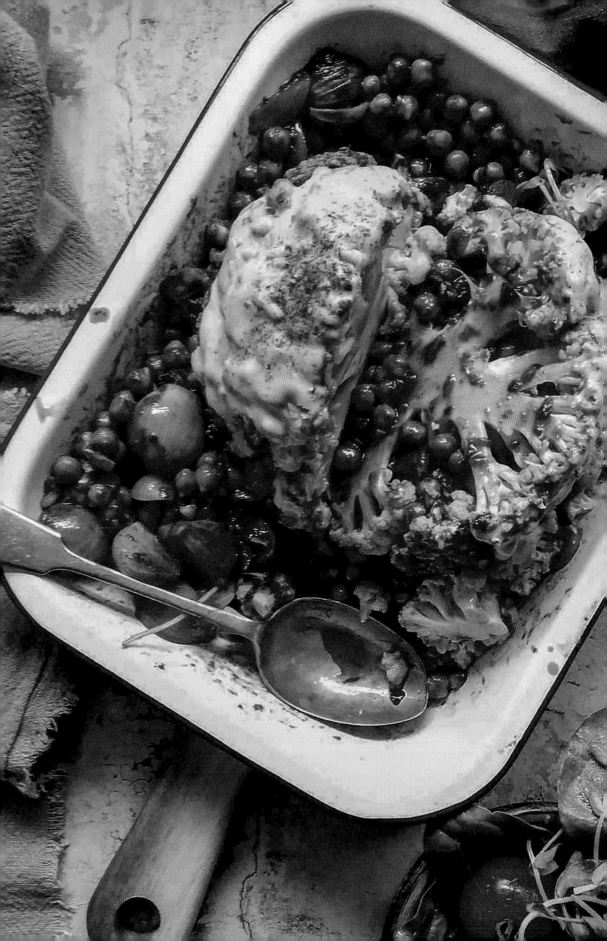

Roasted Harissa Cauliflower Head with Cheese Sauce

Serves 4

Ingredients

- 1 Whole cauliflower
- 8-12 tsp Harissa paste
- 3 Garlic Cloves Finley chopped
- 4 Shallots or 2 onions quartered
- 4-8 Chestnut Mushrooms quartered
- Juice of 1 lemon
- ½ Cup Olive oil (more if you like)
- 1 Tin 400g Chickpeas
- Mixed chopped nuts to sprinkle on top
- 1-2cm size fresh Ginger, peeled and chopped
- ½ Tsp each of Salt, Pepper& Smoked Paprika

Cheese Sauce

- 2 Tbsp plain flour
- 3-4 tbsp olive oil
- Salt & Pepper to taste
- 1 Tsp Smoked paprika
- 2 Cups Soya Milk (more if needed)
- 1 Tsp English mustard
- ½ Tsp Turmeric
- 3-4 Tbsp Nutritional yeast (optional)

Method

1. Preheat the oven 200 fan or 220 conventional ovens. In a bowl mix the (marinade) harissa, oil, garlic, ginger, lemon juice, salt, pepper and paprika and mix well. Remove the leaves from the cauliflower and cut the stem so the cauliflower is able to stand up straight in the baking pan. Place the cauliflower in the centre of an 8 x 10" baking pan and pour the marinade over the cauliflower, keeping some behind to pour over the chickpeas. Rub the marinade over the cauliflower with your hands. Drain the chickpeas and place them in a bowl along with the mushrooms, onions and remainder of the oil and marinade, mix well. Then put the chickpea mixture into the baking pan all round the cauliflower. Put it into the oven and check it after 20 minutes, it should be al dente and not too soft or it will fall apart when cutting into steaks. Whilst the cauliflower is in the oven, make the cheese sauce.

2. Put the oil into a non stick pan, med- to high heat. When the oil has heated add the flour and stir with a whisk, it will turn into a paste. Start adding the milk bit by bit and mix well after adding milk. Once you've added all the milk, simmer to med heat. If you have any lumps, this happens if you add all the milk at once, use a whisk and stir vigorously to get rid of the lumps. Now add the rest of the ingredients in and stir well, taste and season. Simmer for 5 minutes and the sauce will be ready. If it hasn't thickened enough leave it on simmer for a few more minutes, if it's too thick add some more milk to it.

3. When the cauliflower is done, remove from the oven, pour the cheese sauce over the cauliflower and sprinkle with nuts, cut into steaks and serve with the chickpea mixture.

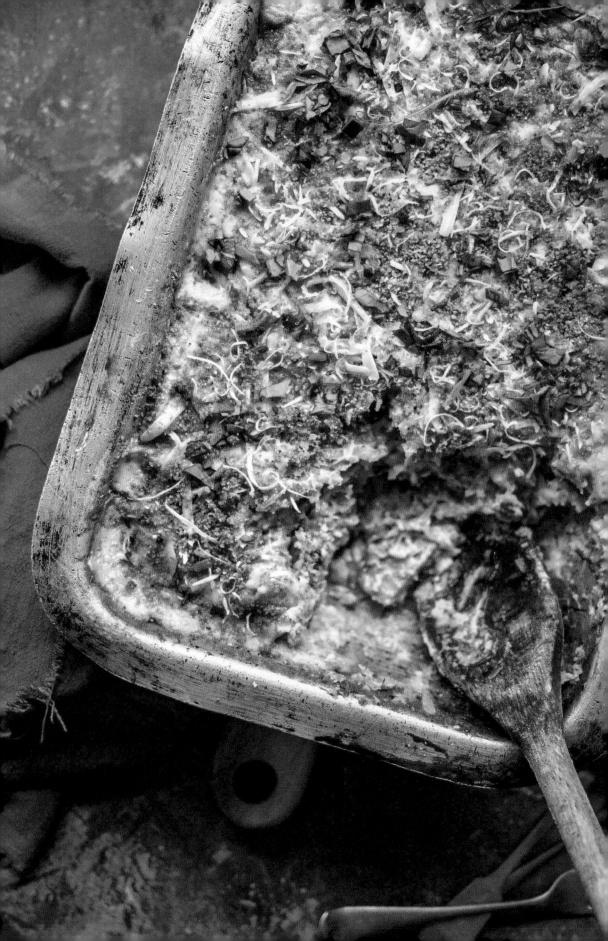

Mixed Root Vegetable Gratin

Serves 6-8 (12x8" Baking tray pan)

Ingredients

- 2x Parsnips roughly chopped
- 1 small-med Swede peeled and roughly chopped
- 4 carrots roughly chopped
- 2 leeks roughly chopped
- 1 Sprig of Rosemary
- 180g cooked chestnuts roughly chopped
- 3 cloves of garlic roughly chopped
- 3Tbsp olive oil
- Grated cheese & breadcrumbs as a topping for the dish

For the white sauce

- 8 Tbsp olive oil
- 7 tbsp plain flour
- 4 cups of soya milk, more if needed
- 1 tsp salt
- 1 tsp pepper
- 1 Tsp English mustard
- 4 tbsp nutritional yeast (optional
- 1 Cup mixed grated cheddar & mozzarella
- Garnish with herb of your choice such as thyme, parsley or mixed herbs.

Method

1. Preheat oven 180 fan or 200 conventional ovens. Place all the vegetables, rosemary, chestnuts & garlic in the baking tray and mix well with the 3 tbsp of oil. In a large pan on a med to high heat, put the 8 tbsp of oil and heat it up. Then add the flour and stir with a whisk, it will turn into a yellow liquid or paste. Start to add the milk bit by bit, stirring in-between every pour to avoid lumps. If lumps form, just whisk vigorously to remove them or use a hand blender. Cook this for 5 minutes; it will start to thicken when you first add the milk. Keep stirring so it doesn't burn. The sauce should be thick but pourable like a cheese sauce, if it's too thick add some more milk, if too thin add some more flour and mix well. Add the salt, pepper, mustard, cheese and nutritional yeast, taste and season. Pour the white sauce into the baking tray and mix well with the vegetables.

2. Place in the oven for 45 min but check after 30 minutes, take it out and give it a good mix. If you find that it has thickened too much, add a bit more milk and mix well. Put it back in the oven for the remainder 15 minutes. Take it out and try some of the vegetables to see if they done. Sprinkle with cheese and breadcrumbs and bake for a further 5- 10 minutes or till the cheese has melted and browned. Garnish with a herb of your choice on top Serve with a side salad or have it as part of a Sunday roast or Christmas lunch.

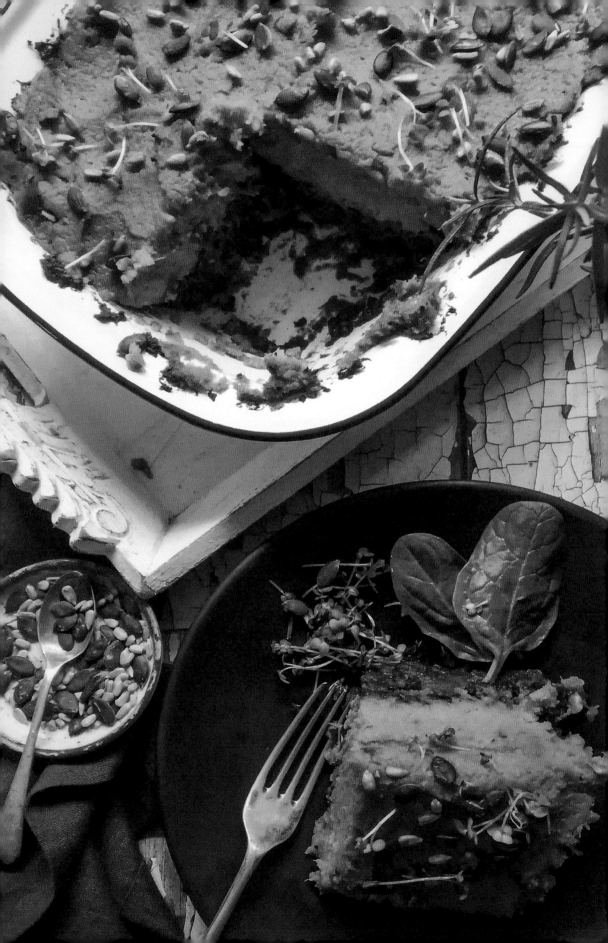

Sweet Potato & Lentil Bake

Serves 4-6

Ingredients

- 3 Large Sweet potatoes peeled and diced
- 1 Large Red Onion Diced
- 4 Garlic Cloves roughly chopped
- 4 Tbsp Olive Oil more if desired
- 1 tin 400g Chopped Tomatoes
- 5 Tbsp Tomato paste
- 2 x 400g cans of cooked brown lentils (can cook from scratch if preferred)
- 1 Tbsp plant butter / margarine
- Salt & pepper to taste
- Sunflower & pumpkin seeds to garnish

Method

1. Boil the potatoes for about 20 min on a med-high heat. Drain the potatoes, add the butter, salt and pepper and mash till smooth, cover and set aside. Preheat the oven to 200 fan or 220 conventional ovens. In a pan on med to high heat add the onions, garlic and oil.

2. Sauté for 2 minutes then add the tomato paste and stir for 1 minute. Add more oil here if needed. Now add the chopped tomatoes and lentils, mix well, taste & season.

3. In a 10 x 7 x 2 "baking pan, pour in the lentil mix and level it out with the back of a spoon. Now add the potato mix, bit by bit and level it out with the spoon.

4. Sprinkle the seeds on top of the mashed potato and bake for 30 minutes or when lightly browned. Serve with a side salad.

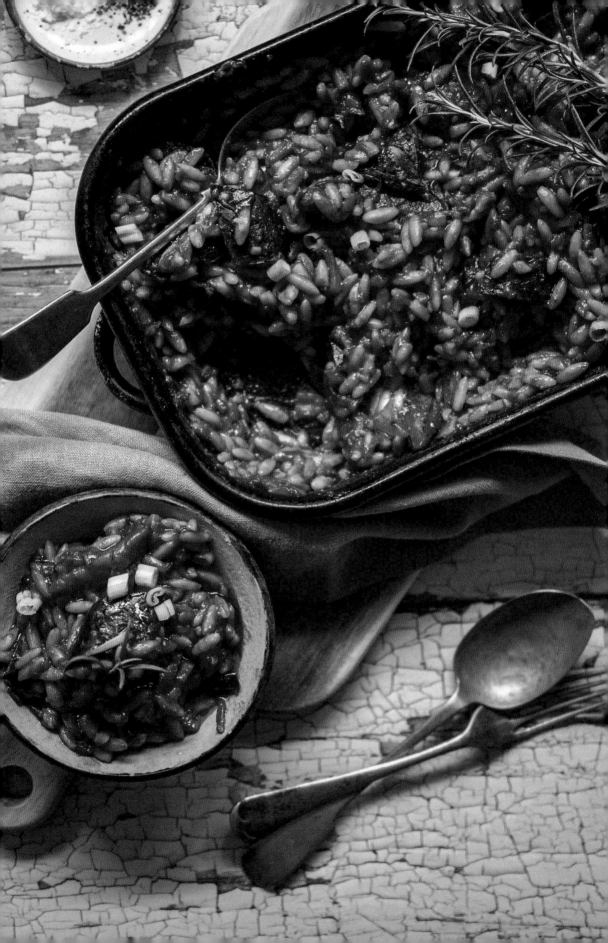

Aubergine & Orzo Oven Bake

Serves 4-6

Ingredients

- 2 Med sized aubergine
- 150-200g uncooked Orzo
- 2 Spring onions finely chopped for garnish
- 2 Shallots sliced
- 1-2 sprigs rosemary
- 1.2 litters water (Not all added at once)
- 200g Tomato Paste
- 400g tin chopped tomatoes
- 3 Cloves garlic
- 6-8 Tbsp olive oil
- Cheese optional
- Salt & Pepper to taste

Method

1. Cut up the aubergine into cubes/ squares with the skin on and rub them with salt to remove moisture, set aside. Preheat oven to 200 Fan or 220 conventional ovens. Put the aubergines, garlic, shallots and 6 Tbsp olive oil in a 13 x 8 x 3 " baking pan, mix well and put in the oven for 20 minutes.

2. In a bowl mix the tomato paste, chopped tomatoes, orzo, rosemary, remainder oil and half of the water. Pour it into the baking tray after the 20 minutes cooking time. Add more water here to cover all the ingredients in the pan. Mix well, cover with foil and place it back in the oven.

3. Turn down the heat to 180 fan or 200 conventional. Take it out after 30 minutes and stir, add more water if it looks dry and in need of more liquid. Put it back in the oven for a further 30 minutes. Take it out and try a piece of aborigine and orzo, if it needs more cooking place it back in the oven with the foil on and if it needs more liquid just add some more water to it. Taste & season.

4. You can add the cheese, if using for the last 5 minutes with the foil removed. Once done sprinkle with spring onion.

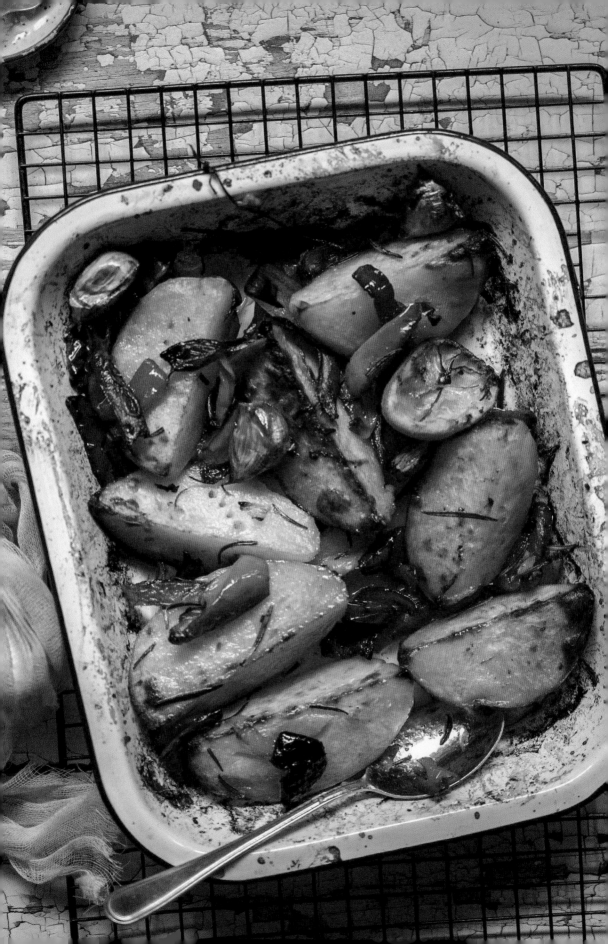

Posh Roast Potatoes

Serves 4-6

Ingredients

- 2 Large potatoes, each cut in 4 wedges
- 1 Green, yellow & Red Pepper roughly chopped
- 2 Sprigs rosemary
- 1 Large red onion roughly chopped
- 3 Garlic cloves whole and skin left on
- ½ cup vegetable oil
- 4 tbsp water
- Salt & Pepper to taste

Method

1. Preheat oven to 200 Fan or 220 Conventional ovens. Place the potatoes, half of the oil and water in a 11x9x2" baking pan and mix well. Put in the oven for 20 minutes.

2. Take out and add the remainder of the ingredients and oil mix well. Turn the oven down to 180 fan or 200 conventional and put back into the oven for an hour.

3. Half way through take it out and give it a good mix so all sides get cooked well. When the hour is up, check the potatoes are done, if not put back for a further 10 minutes at a time until they done.

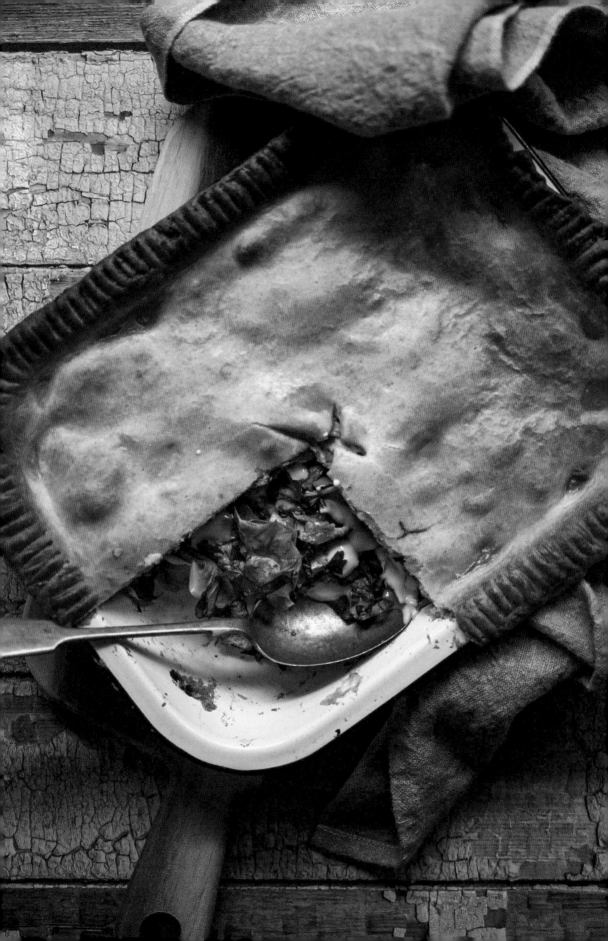

Silken Tofu, Cheese & Vegetables Pie

Serves 4-6

Ingredients

- 2 Packs 375g each Puff Pastry
- 2 Tbsp olive oil
- 3 Garlic Cloves sliced
- 2 -4 Tbsp nutritional yeast optional
- 2 Cups mixed grated cheddar & mozzarella
- 200ml single soya cream
- 1 Tsp English mustard
- ½ Tsp Salt & ½ Tsp ground black pepper
- 1 x Sprig rosemary optional
- 2 Portobello Mushrooms Sliced
- 4 Chestnut Mushrooms sliced
- 70 g baby spinach leaves
- 170 g artichokes from a jar roughly chopped
- 350g silken tofu
- 1 large leek finely sliced
- Milk if needed

Method

1. Using a hand blender or food processor, blend the tofu until smooth, then add the cream, mustard, salt, pepper and nutritional yeast to it and mix well, set aside. Preheat oven to 200 fan 220 conventional ovens. In a pan on a med high heat add oil, mushrooms, garlic & leeks, cook for 5 minutes then add the tofu mixture and cheese and stir for a further 5 minutes. You can add some milk here if it's too thick (consistency should be thick but pourable) and add the rosemary if using. Lightly grease a 12x10x3" baking pan and place one of the puff pastries in the pan making holes in the pastry with a fork. Bake for 10 minutes/ till lightly golden brown. Take it out of the oven and add the ingredients from the pan into the baking dish as a first layer, keeping some behind to add as a top layer. Next layer it with the spinach and then the artichokes. Pour the remaining tofu mixture on top of that and place the second puff pastry over the filling making sure to cover all the edges of the baking pan and use a fork to go round the edges to press the pastry onto the pan, cut off any access pastry. Once you sealed the pie, brush it all over with plant milk and use a sharp knife to cut a cross in the middle for the steam to escape. Turn the oven down to 180 fan or 200 conventional ovens and bake for 15-20 minutes or until pastry is golden brown. You could serve this with some mash and gravy or for a lighter lunch serve with a side salad

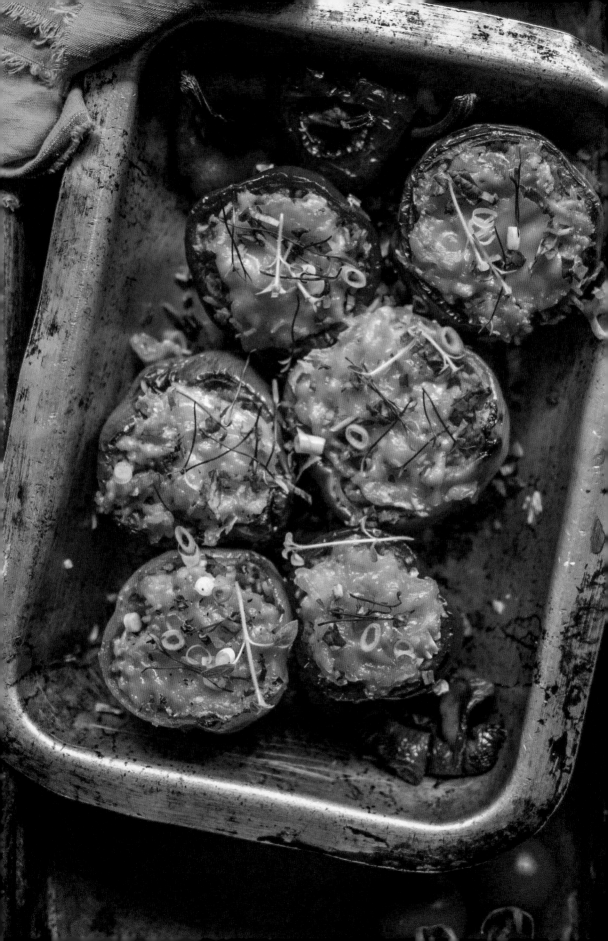

Stuffed Bell Peppers

Serves 4-6

Ingredients

- 6 Mixed colour bell peppers Tops cut off and set aside
- 100g uncooked wild red rice (Plain will also do)
- 4-6 Tbsp olive oil and more for drizzling
- 1Large red onion diced
- 4 Tbsp Tomato paste
- 4 Garlic gloves finely chopped
- 1 Cup dry Soya Mince
- 1 Tin 400g chopped tomatoes
- 1 Tsp fresh/ dry dill (optional)
- 150g of grated cheese, mozzarella and cheddar mixed
- Salt & pepper to taste
- Finely chopped fresh parsley & spring onion to garnish
- Beetroot sprouts to garnish optional
- Juice of ½ a lemon

Method

1. Cook rice to packet instructions but not the full cooking time as it will cook further in the oven. I cooked my rice for 8 min. Drain and set aside. Cut the tops off the peppers and remove the core. Place them in a deep baking try so they can stand up straight.

2. Place them tightly together so they don't fall over. You could use a heatproof ramekin or bowl in the baking tray to help hold the peppers up. Preheat the oven 180 fan or 200 conventional ovens. In a pan on a med-high heat, put 2 tbsp olive oil and the onions, cook for 2 minutes then add the garlic, cook for another minute then add the tomato pure, stir and add more oil to prevent it burning.

3. Stir for another minute and add the chopped tomatoes, stir well, add the soya mince and stir. Simmer for 10 minutes then add the rice & lemon juice to the pan and mix well. If the mixture seems dry add a drop of water, if there is too much liquid, drain it.

4. Fill the peppers with the mixture, put the tops on and put in the oven for 30 – 35 minutes. Remove and feel if the peppers are soft & ready.

5. Take tops off, drizzle olive oil over the peppers and put cheese on top. Put them back in the oven for a further 5 minutes or until the cheese has melted. When they done garnish with parsley, spring onions and beet sprouts. Serve with a side salad.

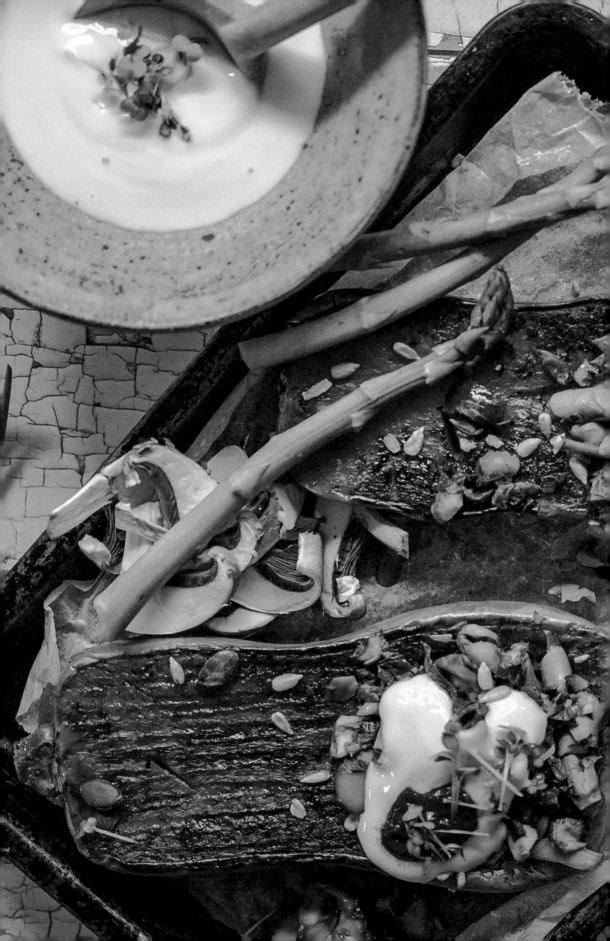

Stuffed Roasted Butternut Squash

Serves 2

Ingredients

- 1 Butternut Squash, Cut in half, skin on and seeds removed
- 70g Baby leaf spinach finely chopped
- 6 Asparagus roughly chopped
- Handful of whole cooked chestnuts roughly chopped
- 2 Portobello mushrooms sliced / roughly chopped
- 4 Spring Onions (1 for Garnish) finely sliced
- 1 cup soya yogurt
- 2-4 Tsp Harissa paste
- 2-4 Tbsp Olive oil
- Juice of 1 lemon optional
- Mixed seeds to sprinkle

Method

1. Preheat the oven to 180 fan 200 conventional ovens. Rub the butternut all over with olive oil. Place them on a baking tray and bake for 35-40 minutes.

2. Half way through baking time, turn the butternut squash over. In a pan on a med – high heat put 2 Tbsp olive oil & spring onions cook for 2 minutes then add the mushrooms and spinach and stir for 1 minute. Add the asparagus & chestnuts and stir for a further 1 minute. Remove from the heat, taste and season.

3. If using lemon add it to the pan now. For the last 10 minutes of cooking time of the butternut squash, fill the butternut with the mixture and put it back into the oven for the remaining 10 minutes.

4. There will be some filling left over which you can serve on the side with the butternut squash. Serve with a dollop of yogurt and harissa paste on top of that. Sprinkle with the spring onions and seeds.

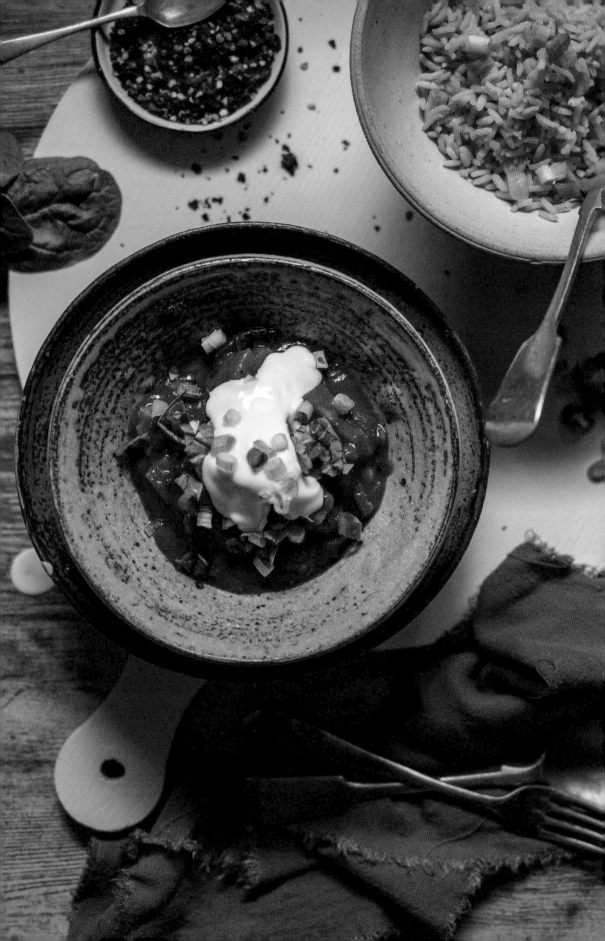

Sweet Potato & Eggplant Coconut Curry

Serves 2

Ingredients

- Ingredients
- 1 Large Sweet Potato diced
- 1 Large eggplant, sliced, salted then diced
- 5 Tbsp Tomato Puree
- 2-4 Tbsp Olive or Sunflower Oil
- 1 Tin 400g of coconut milk
- 3 Spring onions finely chopped (1 to be used for garnish)
- 1 Garlic Clove roughly chopped
- 1-2 cm size fresh ginger, peeled and sliced
- 2-4 Tbsp Soya yogurt for garnish
- 1-2 Tbsp Madras spice (Or any hot spice of choice)
- 2Tsp Turmeric Powder
- 1 Tsp cumin Seeds
- 1 Tsp Hot Paprika
- 70 g baby leaf spinach (optional)
- Salt & pepper to taste

Method

1. Make rice for 2 using packet instructions and add 1 tsp turmeric into the rice water to cook along with the rice. Slice the eggplant lengthways into 4 slices and rub salt on them to absorb all the moisture in the eggplant. Let them rest for a minute or so then cut them into cubes. In a non-stick pan on a med heat, put a dash of oil and panfry the eggplant for 5 minutes and set aside.

2. In a larger pan on a med-high heat, add 2 tbsp oil, garlic, onions and ginger. Sauté for 1 minute then add the remainder turmeric, madras, cumin seeds, paprika, tomato paste and the rest of the oil. Mix well, if you think you need more oil, add some here. Shake the coconut milk can well before opening and add ¾ of it to the larger pan, stir and add the sweet potato and eggplant. Cover and simmer on a med low heat for 20 minutes.

3. Check and stir occasionally. You can add the remainder of the coconut milk if the curry is too thick. Check if the potatoes and eggplant are cooked after the 20 minutes, if not continue to cook checking every 5 minutes. If using the spinach, add it in for the last 5 minutes of cooking time and mix well. Taste & season Serve the curry over the turmeric rice and garnish with a dollop of yogurt and spring onions.

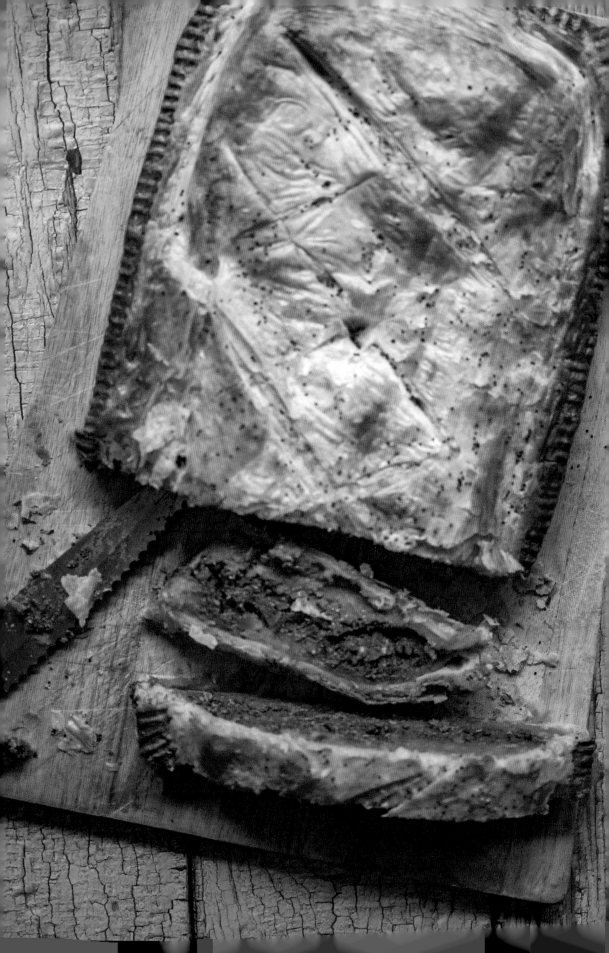

Winter Wellington

 Serves 8-12

Ingredients

(To make a smaller one, half the recipe)

- 2 x 375 g puff pastry
- Soya or any plant milk to brush the pastry
- 1 Large Butternut squash
- 4 Tbsp Olive oil
- 180g cooked chestnuts
- 150g Mixed Nuts
- 1 Red onion roughly chopped
- 2 Garlic cloves whole
- 250g Firm Tofu
- 2 Sprigs rosemary
- 2 ½ Tsp English Mustard
- 1 Tsp Smoked Paprika
- 2 Portobello mushrooms roughly chopped
- 8 Chestnut mushrooms roughly chopped
- 2-4 Slices bread for breadcrumbs more if needed
- Salt & Pepper to taste

Method

1. Preheat oven 200 fan 220 conventional ovens. Cut the butternut squash in half, leave the skin on and remove the seeds. Rub the squash with the oil and bake for 30 minutes, check if they done, if not put back for a further 10 minutes or until they soft. Once done, let them cool down and scrape all the squash out, don't use the skin. Mash or use a food processor to blend squash for a smooth constancy. If the mixture is too wet and not firm enough to hold shape, add some breadcrumbs to it till you get the correct consistency that will hold well in the wellington, set aside. Turn the oven down to 180 fan 200 conventional ovens.

2. In a food processor add the nuts and chestnuts and pulse till they roughly chopped and not smoothed as you want a bit of texture, once chopped set aside. Now put the remainder of the ingredients except the squash mix, nut mix and breadcrumbs into the food processor and mix till well combined ,transfer to a pan on a high heat and cook for 5-8 minutes to remove the moisture of the mushrooms, stirring every minute or so. When done transfer it to a bowl, add the nut mixture and combine well. Check the consistency and add breadcrumbs till mixture is firm to hold shape but not too much breadcrumbs to dry it out, set aside to cool. Line a 15 x 10 "baking pan with baking parchment and place one of the puff pastries on top of the parchment as your bottom part of the wellington. Now add a layer of the cooled down squash mix (1/2 of it) onto the pastry, leaving 1-2 cm free all round the edges so you can seal both pastries together once done. Next layer, the cooled down mushroom mix, place on top of the squash layer, level it out and use your hands to form a nice firm and curved shape, making sure it is well pressed and neat. Take the remainder of the squash mix and place it on top of that, again using your hands to press it all together. Now that it's all pressed and neat, cover it with the second pastry. Use your hands to go over the pastry to smooth it over the filling and tuck it in the sides so there are no air gaps. Before sealing the top to the bottom, brush the bottom pastry with milk to act as a glue to hold the pastries together. Using a fork to go round the edges to seal the pastries further and cut off any access pastry. Brush the entire wellington with milk and use a knife to make diagonal lines over the pastry without cutting into it, just lightly cutting for decoration purposes. In the centre of the wellington, use a sharp knife to cut a cross into the pastry for the steam to escape. Bake for 30 minutes or until golden brown.

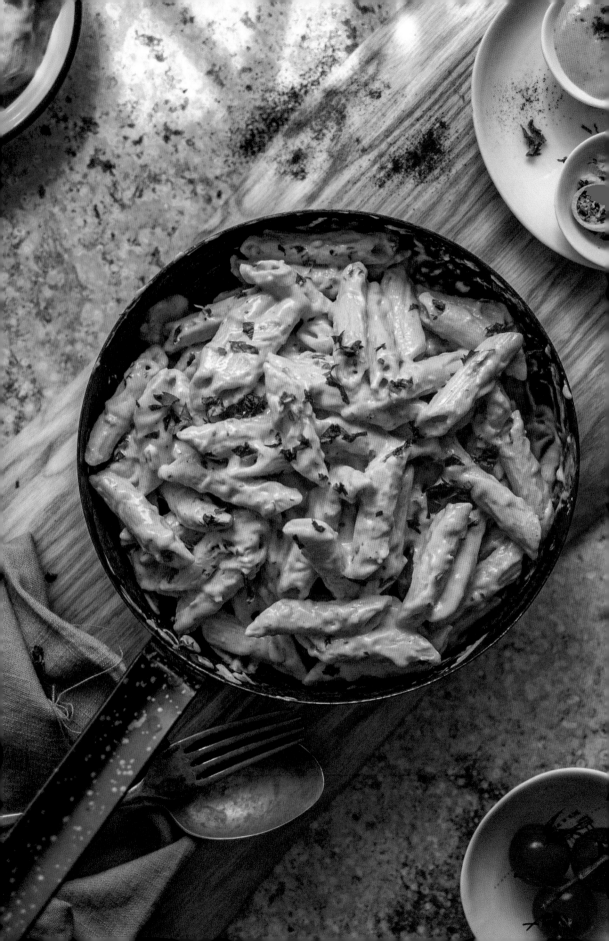

Pasta

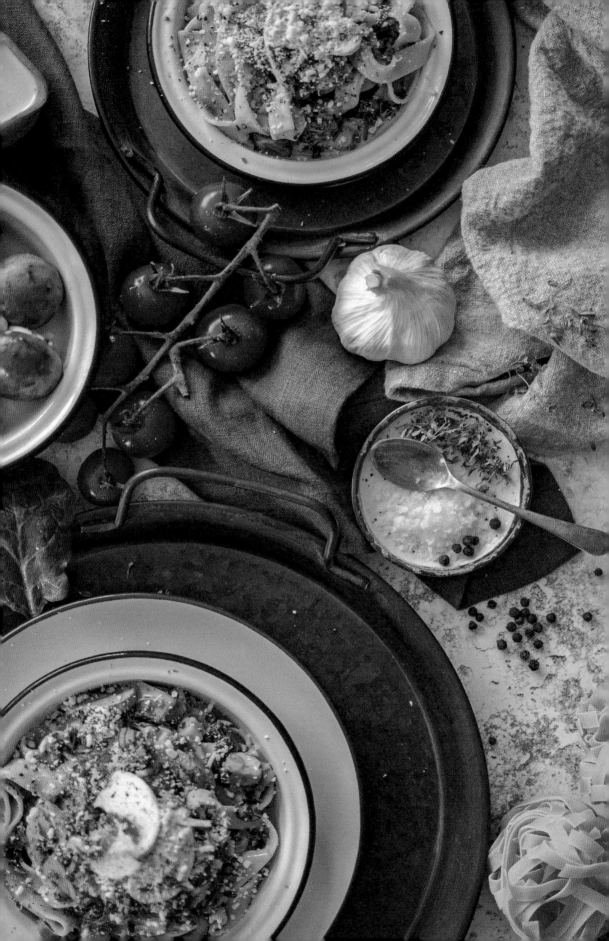

Garlic Mushrooms & Spinach Fettuccini Pasta

Serves 2-3

Ingredients

- 1x Pack Fettuccini Pasta
- 300g Chestnut Mushrooms Sliced
- 6 Garlic Cloves roughly chopped
- 2 x 250g Soya Single Cream cartons
- 125g Baby Spinach Leaves
- 2 Tbsp Olive Oil
- Salt & pepper to taste (This dish is great with a lot of black pepper)
- Parmesan Cheese to serve

Method

1. Make the pasta to the packet instructions.

2. In a pan on a med to high heat, fry the mushrooms and garlic with the olive oil for 6-8 minutes.

3. Add the cream and continue to cook for a further 5 minutes then add the spinach and turn off the heat, Mix it well and season. Serve with parmesan cheese.

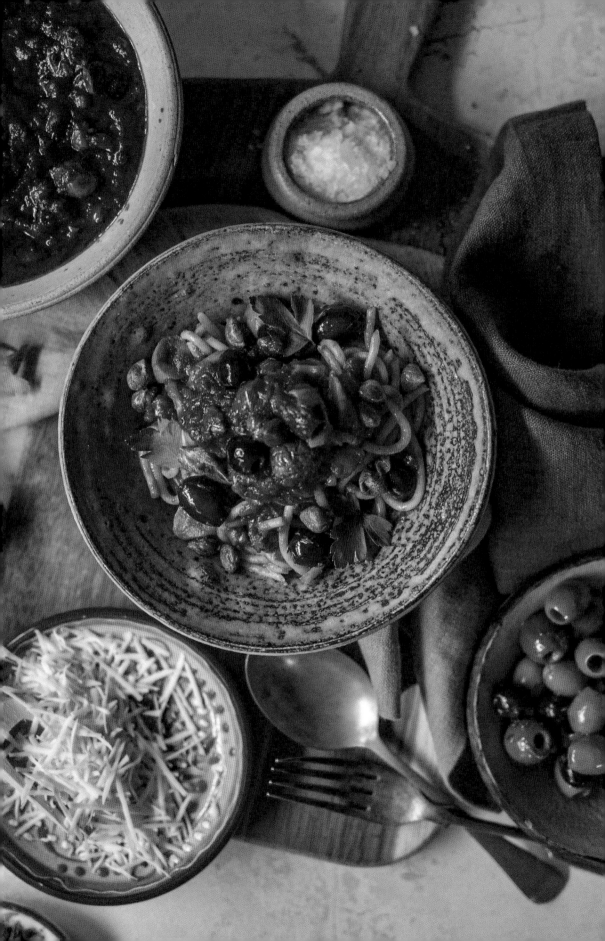

Arribiata Spaghetti

Serves 2

Ingredients

- Spaghetti enough for 2
- 2 Garlic cloves roughly chopped
- ½ Red Onion diced
- 3 Tbsp Tomato paste
- 1 Tbsp Olive Oil
- 400g tin chopped tomatoes
- 150g mixed & pitted olives roughly chopped
- 50g capers

Method

1. Make spaghetti to packet instructions.

2. In a pan on a med high heat, put the oil, capers, onions and garlic and sauté for 1-2 minutes.

3. Add the tomato puree and olives, stir well for a minute, add more oil here if you like. Pour the tin tomatoes in, stir and simmer for 10- 15 minutes.

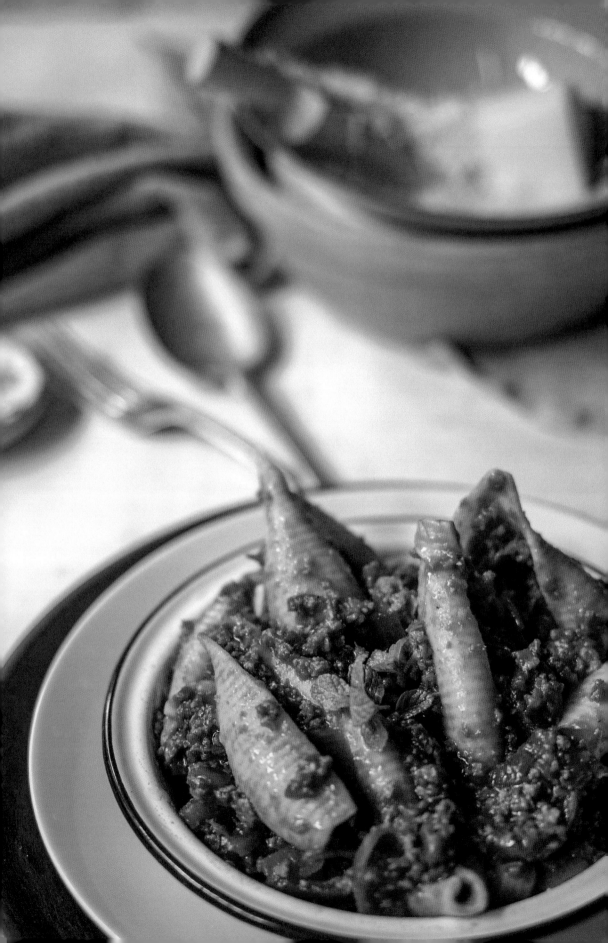

Soya Bolognaise Shells

Serves 2-3

Ingredients

- 1 x Pack of Pasta shells
- 2-6 Tbsp Olive oil
- 1 Red Onion Diced
- 2 Garlic Cloves roughly chopped
- 1 Can 400g Chopped Tomatoes
- Salt & Pepper to taste
- 6 Tbsp Tomato Paste
- 1 Cup Dry Soya Mince
- ½-1 tsp Dried or Fresh oregano or Thyme to garnish
- Grated Cheddar or parmesan Cheese
- Water as needed

Method

1. Make pasta to packet instructions.

2. In a pan on med- high heat, add 2 tbsp olive oil, onions & garlic, sauté for 2-3 minutes. Then add the tomato puree and sauté for another minute add more oil here if needed.

3. Simmer to a med-low heat and add the tin of chopped tomatoes and soya mince. Mix it well and see if you need to add any water to it, the soya mince will swell but only a little bit.

4. You can also add the remainder oil in now. Simmer to a low heat for 15 minutes with the lid on. Check and stir every 5 minutes or so.

5. If it's too thick, just add some more water, making sure the ratio of mince and liquid is balanced.

6. Turn the heat off and add the herb of your choice and stir. Serve with grated cheese of your choice.

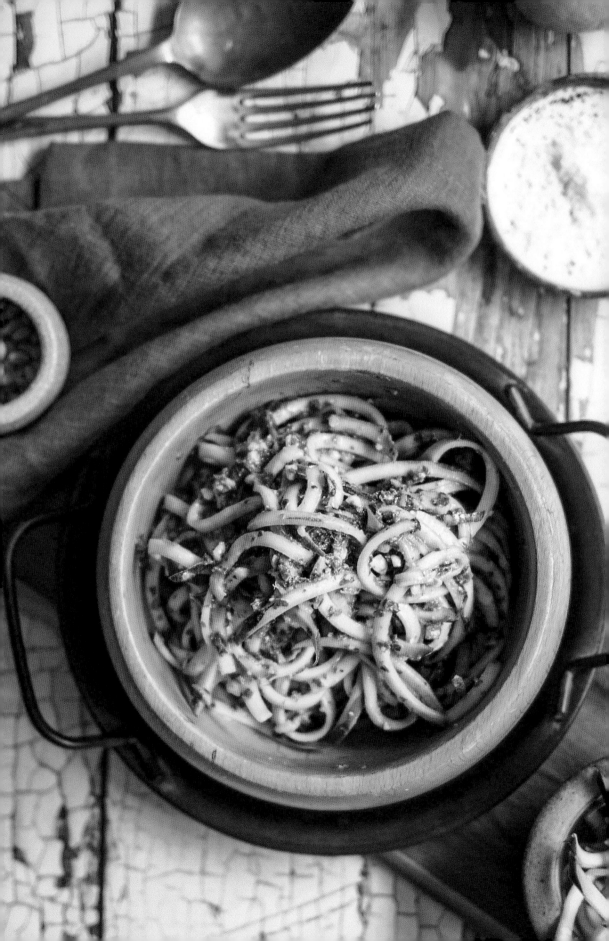

Courgetti Spaghetti with Kale & Spinach Pesto

Serves 2-4

Ingredients

For the Kale & Spinach Pesto

- 180g chopped kale
- 125g baby leaf spinach
- ½ cup mixed chopped nuts
- Handful of pine nuts
- 4 large garlic cloves
- 1 cup Olive Oil
- ½ cup vegetable Oil
- 4 Tbsp Nutritional Yeast (Optional)
- Juice of 1 large Lemon
- Salt and pepper to taste

For the Pasta

- 2 – 4 courgettes (1 per Person)

Method

1. Firstly put nuts, not the pine nuts into a food processor and blitz till roughly chopped for a nice texture & leave them in the processor. Then add the kale and blitz again, add some of the olive oil here to allow it to mix well and until it's a nice fine texture. Now add the rest of the ingredients except the pine nuts and hold back the ½ cup of sunflower oil which you can add right at the end if needed. Mix well in the processor to your desired texture, taste and season with salt & pepper, add the pine nuts and use the pulse on the processor for a final mix.

2. Using a spiralizer, spiralize the amount of courgettes needed. You can mix it with the pesto in a large bowl or you can plate up the courgette spaghetti and put the pesto on top and serve with some pine nuts sprinkled over the dish. This dish can be eaten hot or cold. If you prefer it hot, mix the courgette and pesto before placing in a pan and heat up for 5 minutes on a med to high heat. It's very nutritious eaten raw.

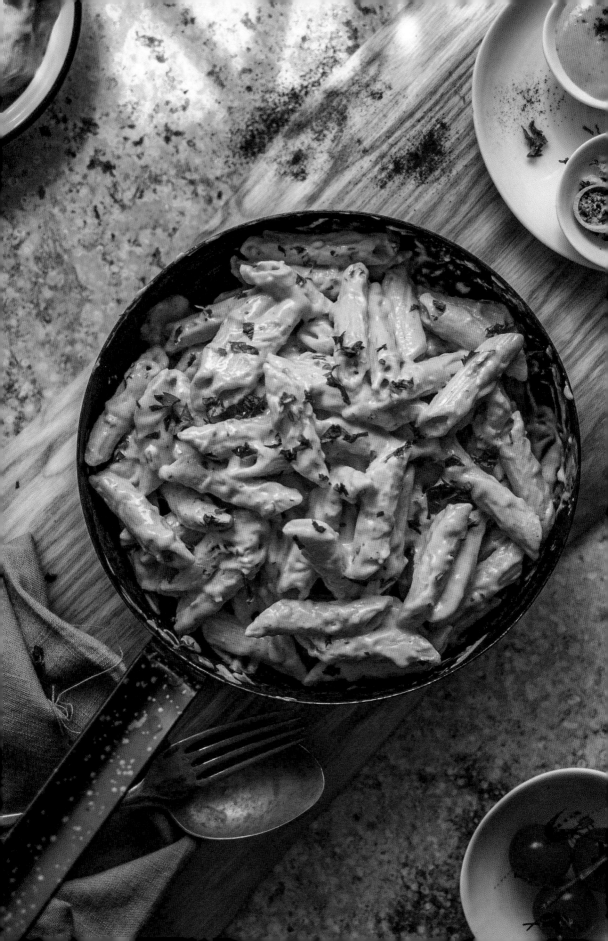

Mac & Cheese

Serves 4-6

Ingredients

- 500g Penne Pasta
- 1/3 Cup Vegetable Oil
- 8 Tbsp Plain Flour
- 6 Cups Soya Milk
- 2 Tsp Smoked Paprika
- 4-6 Tbsp Nutritional Yeast (Optional, adds a cheese & nutty flavour)
- 1 ½ Tsp English Mustard
- 2 Tsp Salt
- Pepper to taste
- 2 ½ Tsp Turmeric Powder
- 1 Cup grated cheddar optional
- 2 Tbsp Red Wine Vinegar optional
- Parsley for garnish optional

Method

1. Make the pasta according to packet instructions. Whilst waiting for the pasta start making the cheese sauce. In a pan, heat up the oil on a med-high heat. Add the flour and stir; it will turn into a yellow paste.

2. Pour the milk in bit by bit stirring after each pour with a whisk to avoid lumps. Once all the milk has been used up simmer and add the remainder ingredients and keep stirring every minute or so, it will start to thicken. If you have lumps in the sauce, use a hand whisk and stir vigorously to get rid of the lumps.

3. You can also use a hand blender to remove lumps and also get a smoother sauce. If the sauce is too thick you can add some extra milk, if too thin add a Tbsp of flour, mix well and let it simmer for a further 5 minutes to cook the flour.

4. When the pasta is ready, drain it and transfer it into a larger pot so you can pour the cheese sauce over it and mix it well. You can sprinkle with parsley if using and extra grated cheese on top if you like.

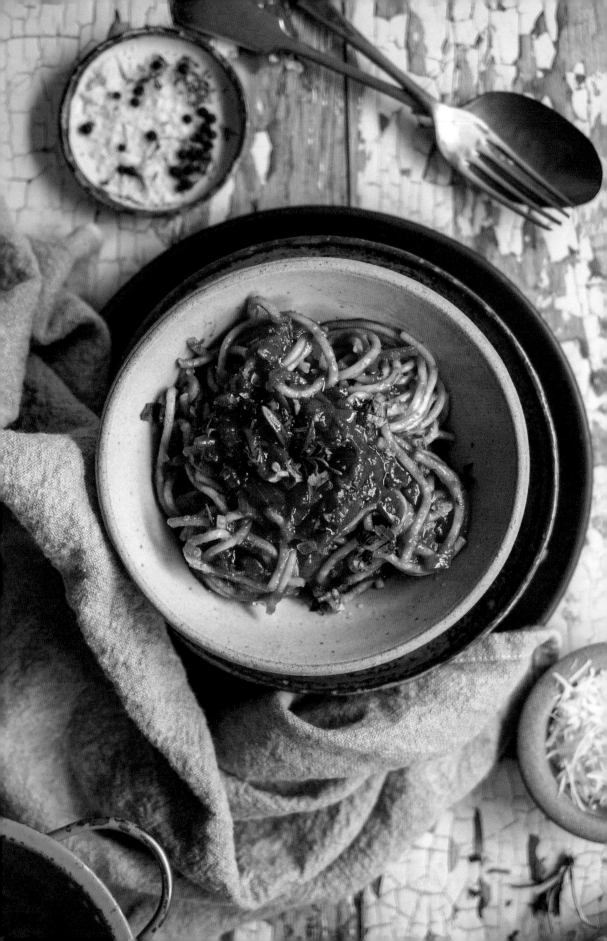

Napolitana Spaghetti

Serves 2

Ingredients

- ½ Packet Spaghetti / enough for 2
- 2 Garlic cloves roughly chopped
- ½ Red onion diced
- 3 Tbsp Tomato Pure
- 400g tin of chopped tomatoes
- 2 Tbsp Olive Oil
- Salt & Pepper to taste
- ½ tsp dry herb of choice optional
- Cheese for topping optional

Method

1. Make spaghetti to packet instructions.

2. In a pan on a med high heat, put the oil, onions and garlic and sauté for 1-2 minutes. Add the tomato puree and stir well for a minute, add more oil here if you like. Pour the tin tomatoes in, stir and simmer for 5- 8 minutes.

3. If using herbs add them in the last minute of cooking, taste & season. Serve on top of the spaghetti and sprinkle some cheese over it if using.

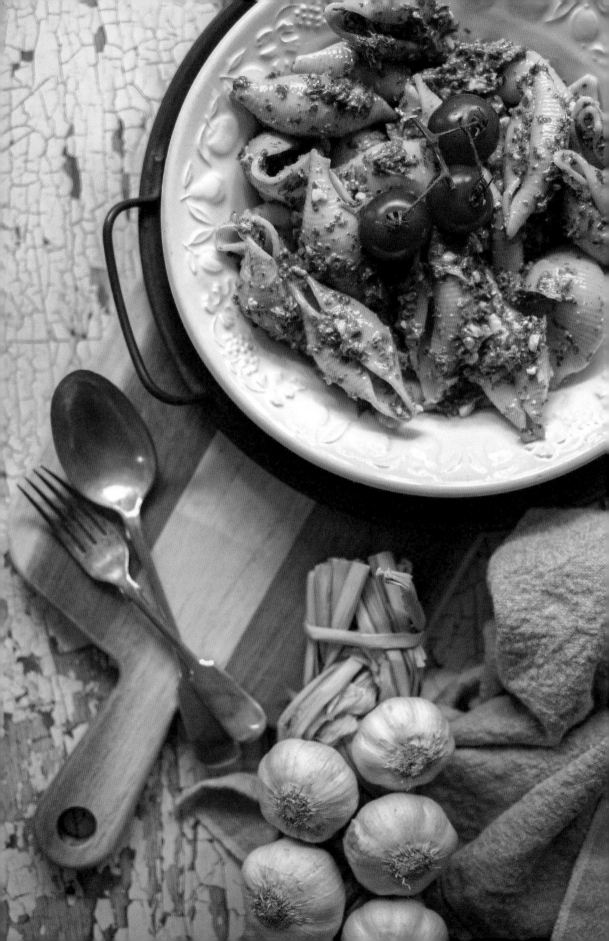

Kale & Spinach Pesto Pasta Shells

Serves 4

Ingredients

- Pasta shells enough for 4
- 180g chopped kale
- 125g baby leaf spinach
- ½ cup mixed chopped nuts
- Handful of pine nuts
- 4 large garlic cloves
- 1 cup Olive Oil
- ½ cup vegetable Oil
- 4 Tbsp Nutritional Yeast (Optional)
- Juice of 1 large Lemon
- Salt and pepper to taste
- Parmesan optional

Method

1. Make pasta to packet instructions.

2. To make the pesto, put nuts, not the pine nuts into a food processor and blitz till roughly chopped for a nice texture & leave them in the processor. Then add the kale and blitz again, add some of the olive oil here to allow it to mix well and until it's a nice fine texture.

3. Now add the rest of the ingredients except the pine nuts and hold back ½ cup of sunflower oil which you can add right at the end if needed. Mix well in the processor to your desired texture, taste and season with salt & pepper, add the pine nuts and use the pulse on the processor for a final mix.

4. To serve, you can add the pesto with the pasta in a larger pot and mix well. To keep all the nutrients, don't heat the pesto. If you prefer the pesto to be warm then heat it up in a pan before mixing with the pasta shells. Sprinkle with parmesan.

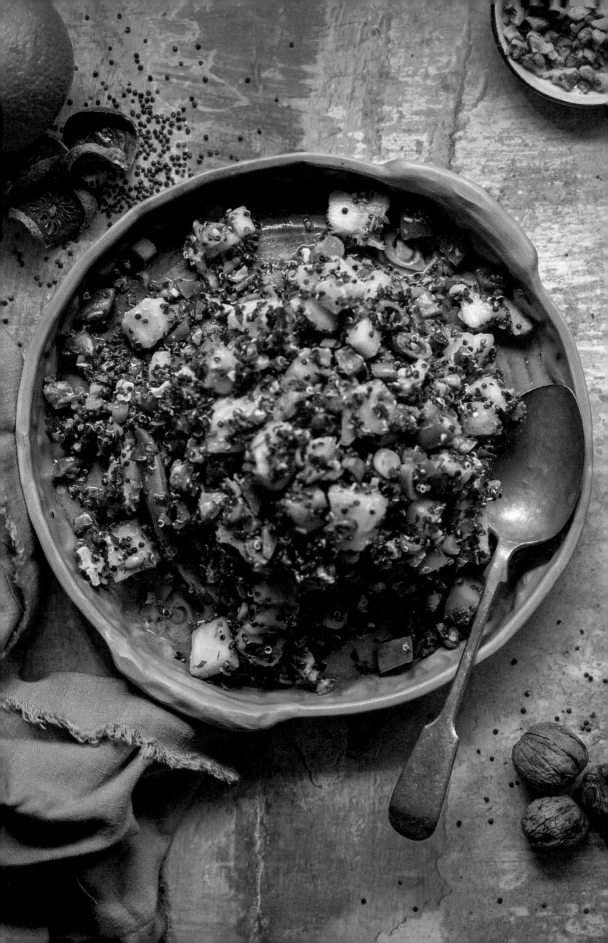

Salads

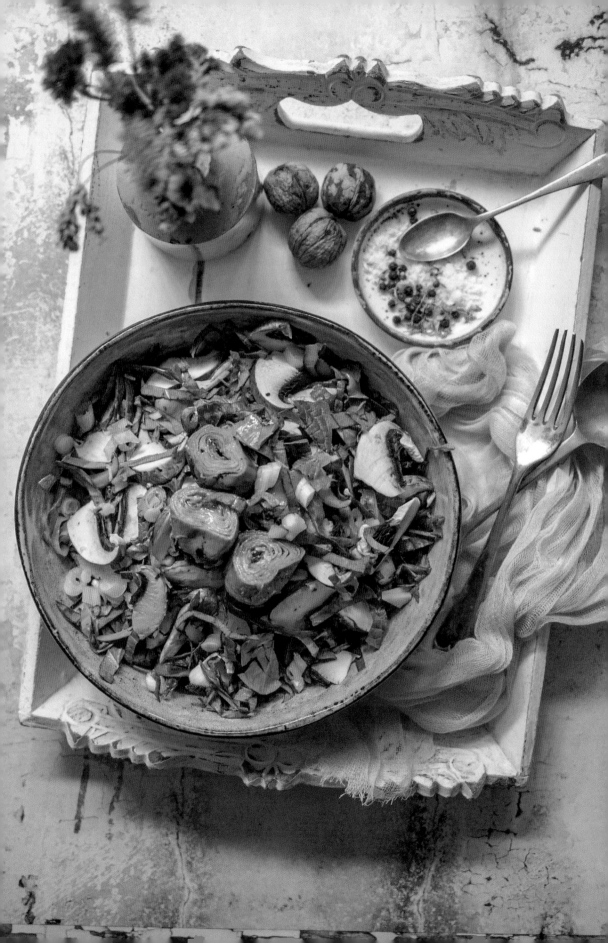

Artichoke, Mushroom & Spinach Salad

Serves 2-4

Ingredients

- 3-4 Large Portobello Mushrooms raw & sliced
- 150g Baby leaf Spinach, raw & finely chopped
- 3 Spring Onions Finley Chopped
- 150g Artichokes from a jar roughly chopped
- 4 Tbsp Olive Oil
- Juice of 1 Lemon

Method

1. Mix all ingredients into a salad bowl then add the lemon juice & oil.
2. Mix well, taste and season.

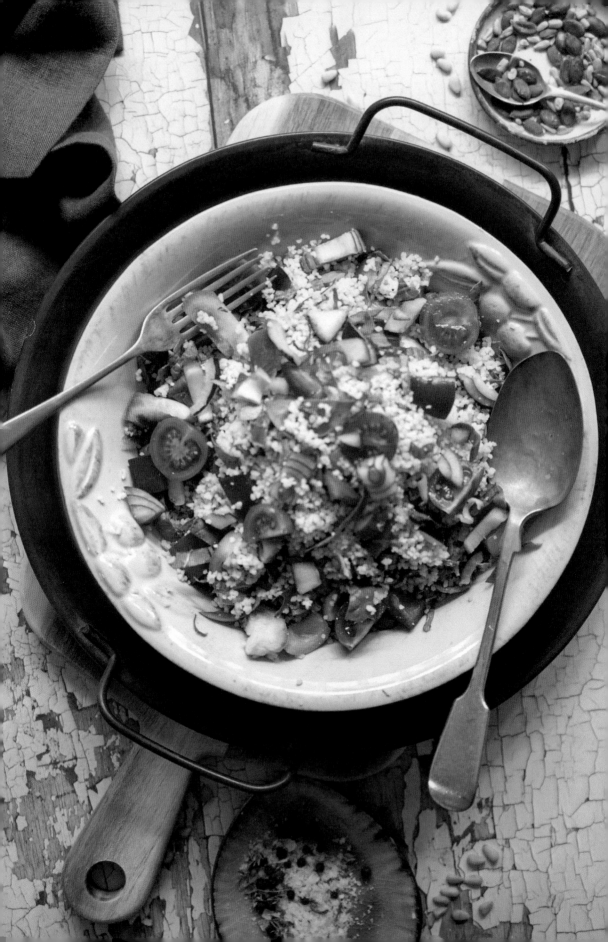

Couscous Salad

Serves 4-6 Serve hot or cold

Ingredients

- 1 Cup couscous
- 1 & ½ cup hot water
- 300g cherry tomatoes, whole or cut in half/ quartered
- 1 Green pepper diced
- 1 Red Pepper diced
- 1 Yellow Pepper diced
- 1 Large red onion diced
- 4 Tbsp Olive oil
- Juice of 1 lemon
- 1 Tsp Salt & ½ Tsp Pepper
- 150g raw baby spinach leaves finely chopped

Method

1. Put the couscous in a bowl add salt, pepper, oil, lemon juice and the hot water. Set aside, don't stir it. Wait for at least 2 minutes before scraping it out of the bowl with a fork into another bowl.

2. If you use a spoon and over stir, the couscous will get stuck together and form big lumps.

3. Once you've carefully scrapped out the couscous into another bowl, add the remainder ingredients and mix gently with your hands. Taste and add more seasoning if needed.

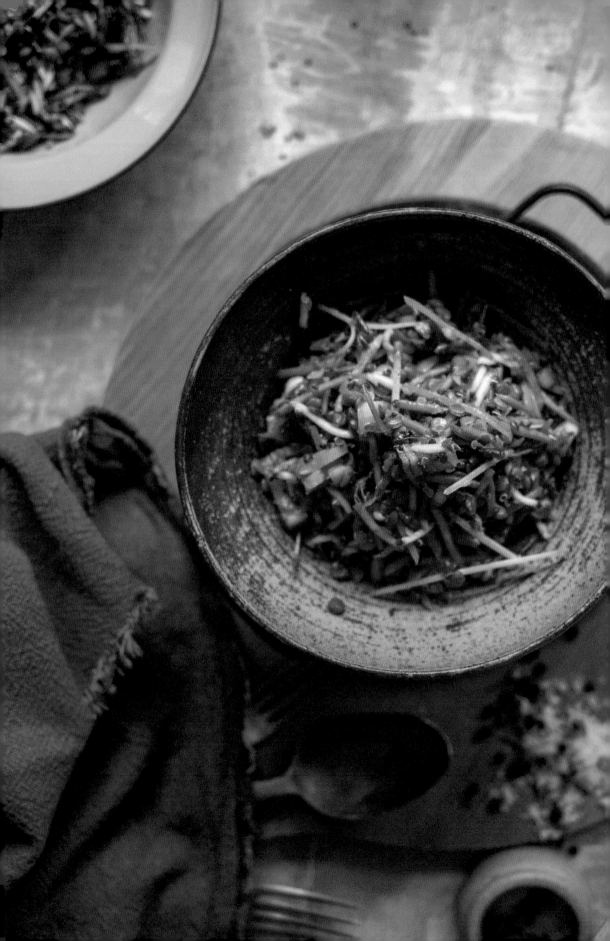

Quinoa & Lentil Salad

Serves 4

Ingredients

- 1 Cup uncooked brown Lentils
- ¼ cup uncooked red quinoa
- 2 Med carrots grated or shredded
- 1 med courgette grated or shredded
- Bunch of pea shoots or other preferred sprouts
- 2 Spring Onions Finely Chopped
- 1 Red onion finely diced
- 1-2 Tbsp Apple cider vinegar
- 4-6 Tbsp Olive oil
- Juice of 1 lemon
- Salt & Pepper to taste

Method

1. Rinse quinoa well before cooking. Cook lentils and quinoa to packet instructions.

2. Once lentils and quinoa are cooked, rinse under cold water and drain well.

3. In a large bowl mix all the ingredients together adding half the oil and vinegar taste and add the remainder if needed and season with salt and pepper.

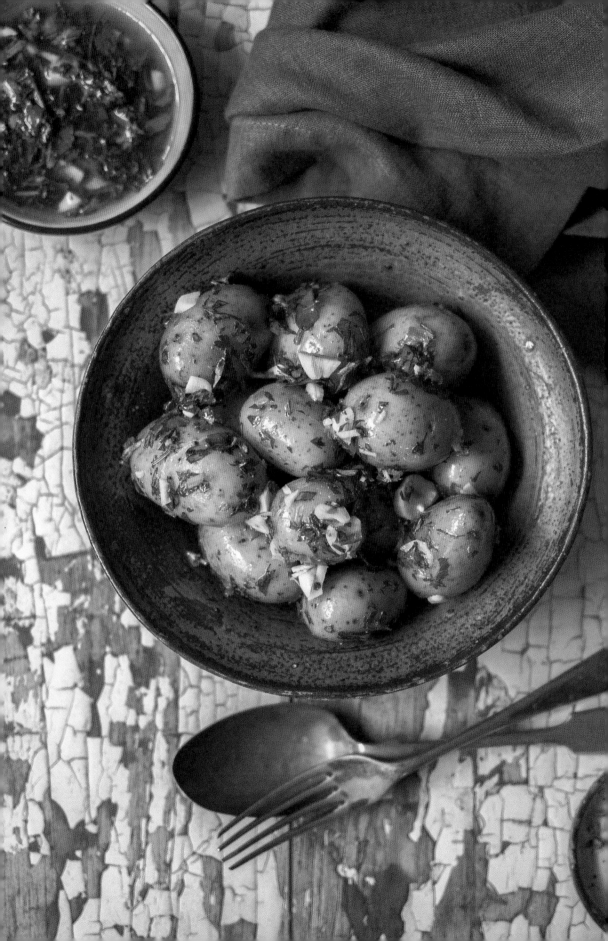

Garlic & Parsley New Potatoes Salad

Serves 2-4

Ingredients

- 500g new potatoes with skin on
- 3-4 Tbsp Olive oil
- Juice of ½ a lemon
- 3 Garlic Cloves finely chopped
- ½ bunch or 10g Parsley finely chopped
- Salt & Pepper to taste

Method

1. Boil the potatoes with skin on for 25-30 minutes on a med-high heat.

2. Drain and rinse with cold water to cool the potatoes down.

3. Transfer to a salad bowl and mix the remainder ingredients together, taste and season.

4. If you think you need more oil, add it now.

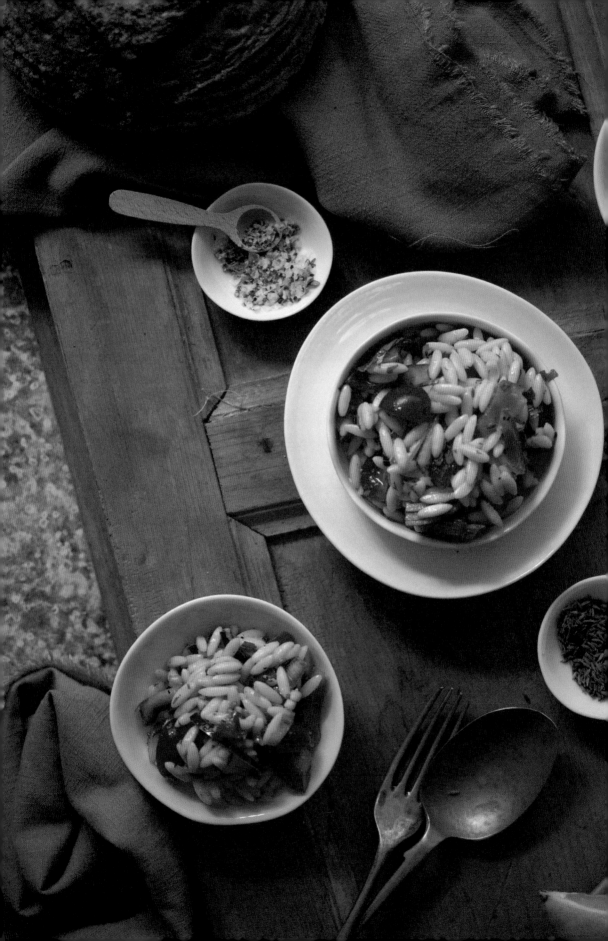

Orzo Salad

Serves 2-4

Ingredients

- 240g uncooked Orzo
- Salt & Pepper to taste
- 2 Tsp Turmeric Powder
- 220g Cherry Tomatoes quartered
- Juice of 1 lemon
- 1 green pepper finely chopped
- 1 red onion diced
- Handful of parsley finely chopped
- 4 tbsp olive oil
- 2 tsp cumin seeds

Method

1. Cook orzo to packet instructions and add the turmeric to the water to dye the orzo yellow.

2. Once the orzo is done, rinse it with cold water to cool it down.

3. Drain well and transfer to a salad bowl.

4. Mix the remainder of the ingredients to the bowl, taste and season.

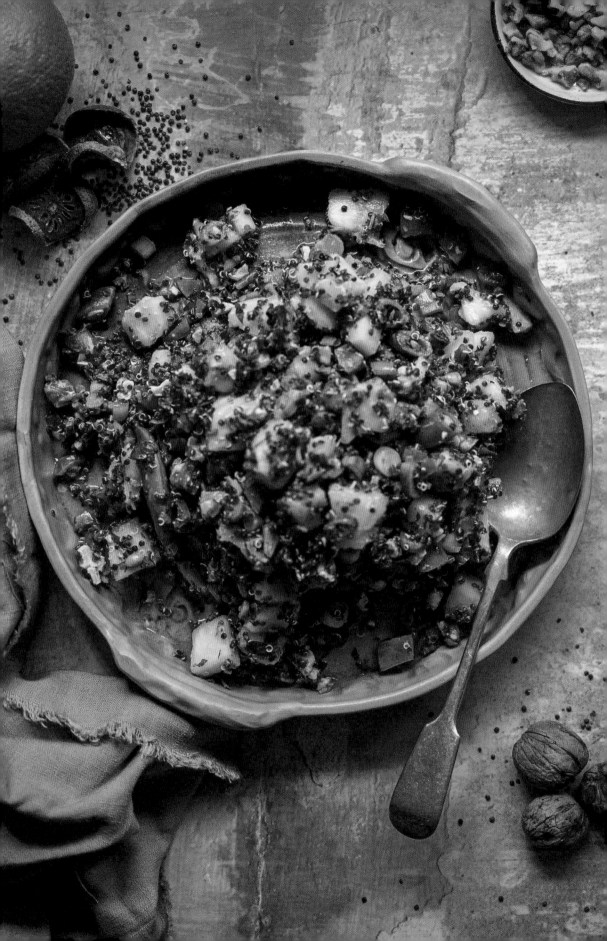

Red Quinoa & Pineapple Salad

Serves 4

Ingredients

- ½ cup uncooked red quinoa
- ½ cup walnuts chopped
- 150g raw sugar snaps chopped
- 2 spring onions finely chopped
- 1 small – med pineapple diced
- Handful of parsley or basil finely chopped
- Juice of 1 orange
- Juice of 1 lemon
- Pinch of salt
- 4-6 Tbsp Olive oil

Method

1. Cook quinoa to packet instructions but rinse well before cooking.

2. Cut up all your fruit and vegetables. Once the quinoa is ready, rinse under cold water and drain well.

3. In a salad bowl, mix all the ingredients together and enjoy x

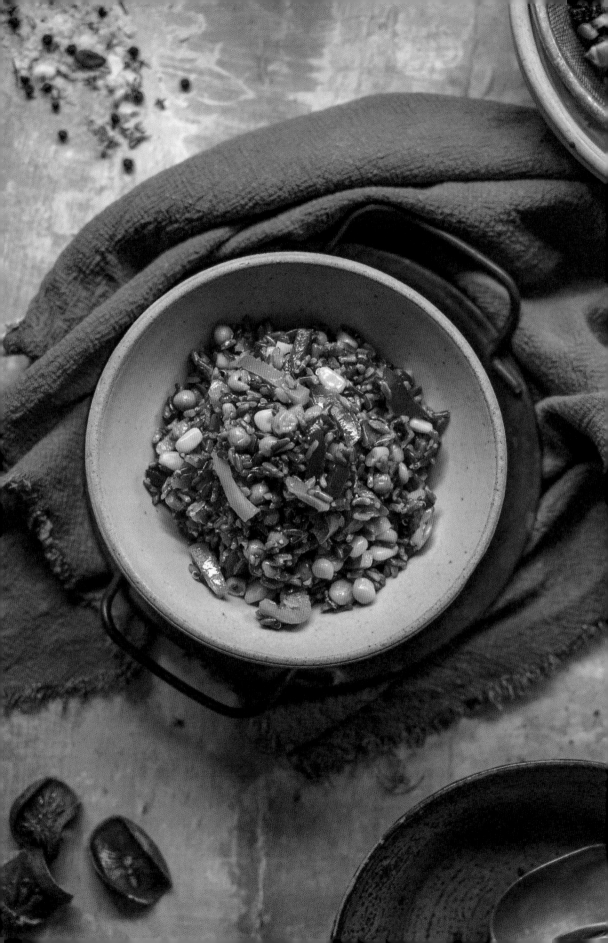

Wild Red Rice Salad

Serves 2

Ingredients

- 1 Cup uncooked wild red rice (Can use any if you don't have red rice)
- 60g frozen sweet corn
- 200g frozen mixed peppers
- 50g frozen edamame beans
- 50g frozen green peas
- 1 Tbsp Apple cider vinegar
- 1-3 Tbsp Olive oil
- Salt and pepper to taste

Method

1. Cook the rice to packet instructions. For the last 10 minutes of the rice cooking time, add the edamame beans to the rice and after 4 minutes add the sweet corn. Let that cook for a further 2 minutes then add the peppers to cook for the next 2 minutes and finally add the peas for the last 2 minutes.

2. If you need to add some hot water to the rice once you add the vegetables, then do so and you can drain the access water after everything is cooked. Now drain any water left and add 2 Tbsp of oil to the pan and stir well over a med- high heat for 2 minutes.

3. Remove from the heat and add the vinegar, taste and season. You can add more olive oil now if you need to. I added more vinegar and oil to mine as I really enjoyed it with extra vinegar and oil.

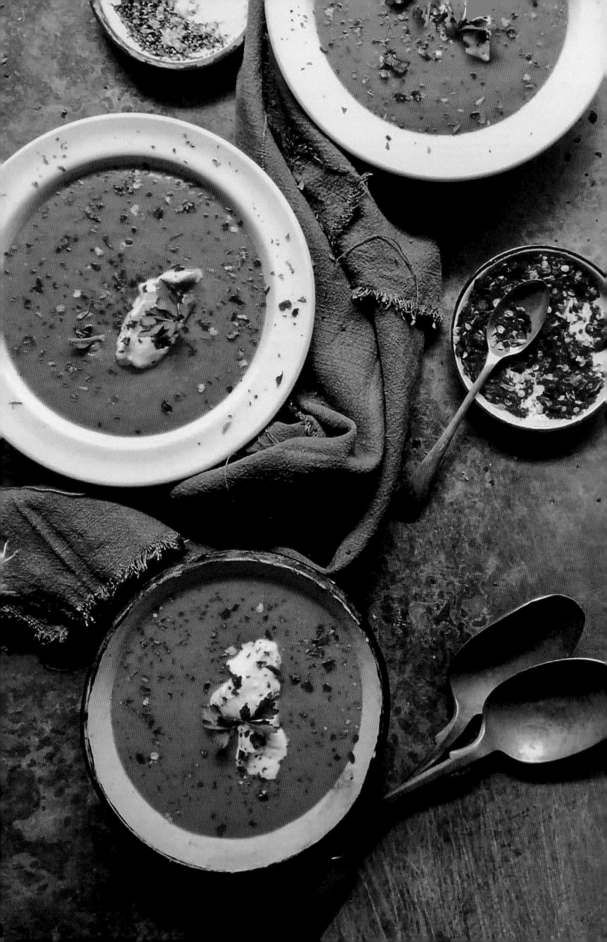

Soups

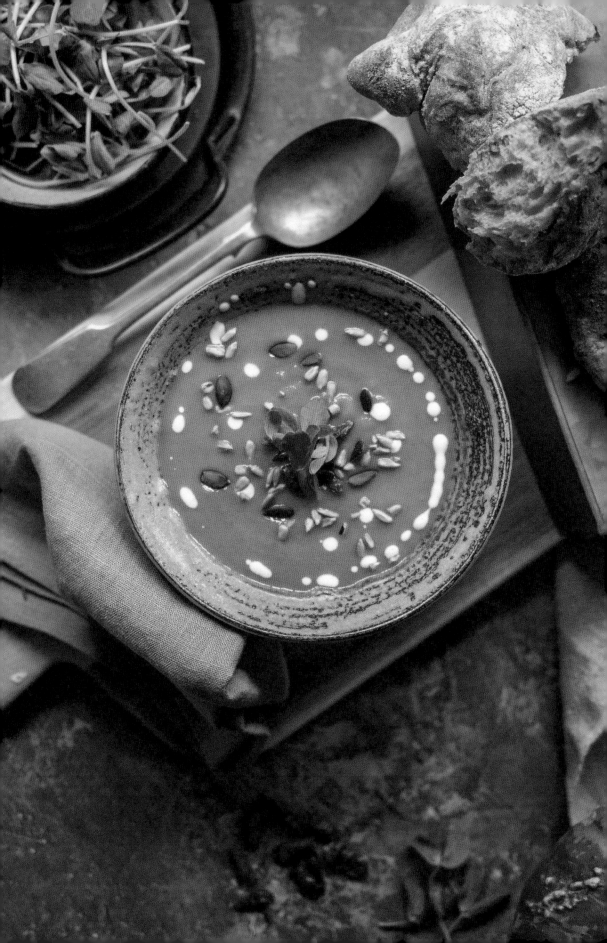

Carrot, Ginger, Sweet Potato & Chilli Soup

Serves 6-8

Ingredients

- 1kg carrots roughly chopped
- 1 Med sweet potato, peeled & roughly chopped
- 30g fresh ginger, peeled and roughly chopped
- 2 garlic cloves roughly chopped
- 1 red onion roughly chopped
- ½ tsp chilli flakes optional
- 2 tbsp olive oil
- Salt & pepper to taste
- 1 litre hot water
- I Tbsp bouillon vegetable stock (mixed in water)

Method

1. Mix the Bouillon into the water. Sauté onions, garlic, ginger in olive oil on high heat for 3 minutes. Add the rest of the ingredients and leave on high heat for 10 minutes then simmer for 20-30 minutes with lid on.

2. Check if the carrots are soft, if so remove from the heat. Using a hand blender, blend till smooth.

3. You can pour cream over the soup when serving and sprinkle some seeds and more chilli flakes if you like chillies.

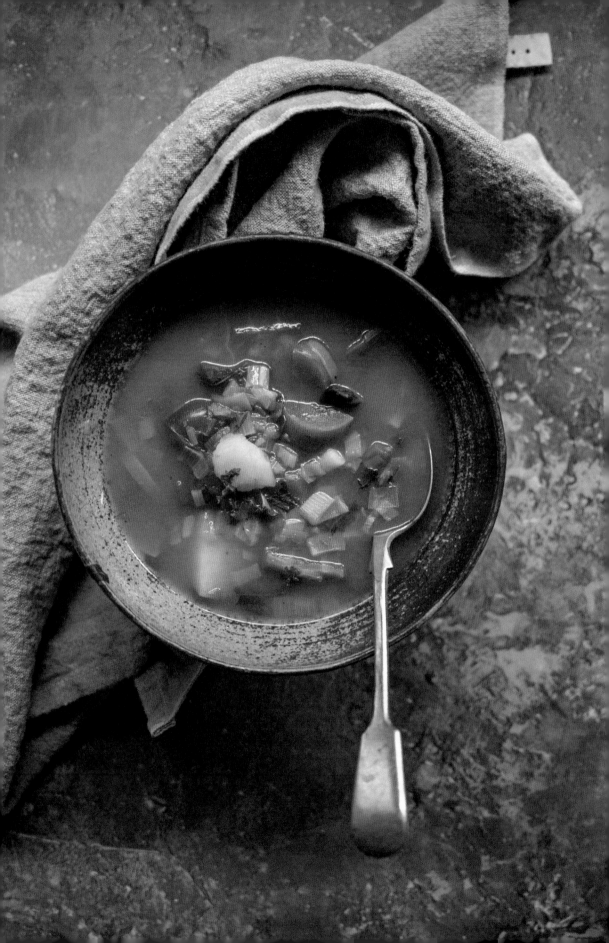

Chunky Vegetable Soup

Serves 4-6

Ingredients

- 2 tbsp olive oil
- 5 celery sticks roughly chopped
- 1 large Leek finely sliced
- 4 med carrots roughly chopped
- 2 large potatoes roughly chopped, skin left on or peeled off
- 100-150g baby spinach leaves roughly chopped
- 70 g spring greens roughly chopped
- 50g kale fine to roughly chopped
- 2 tbsp bouillon vegetable stock
- 500ml hot water for stock
- Salt and pepper to taste

Method

1. Mix the bouillon into the hot water and set aside. Sauté celery, leek and oil on a med to high heat for 3 min then add the remaining ingredients except the spinach and turn down to med heat.

2. Put the lid on the pot and check after 30 min, if the potatoes and carrots are soft, it's done,

3. if not, simmer and check every 10 minutes. Add the spinach for the last 5 min of cooking. Add salt and pepper.

4. You can serve this as a chunky soup or blend it smooth.

Tip :

Cut all your vegetables the same size so that they are all ready at the same time. Keeping the skin on your veggies is a good idea as many of the nutrients are in the skins.

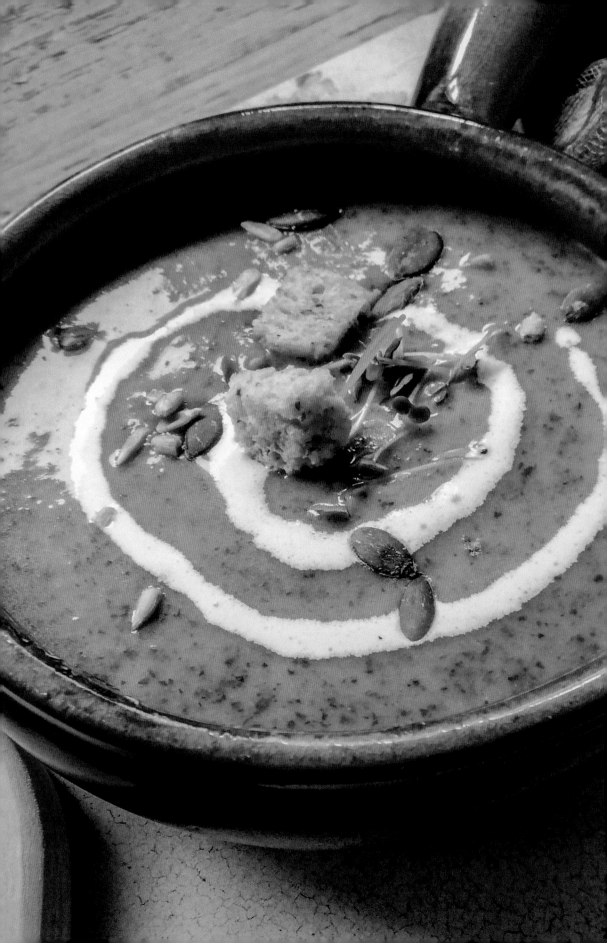

Watercress soup

Serves 4-6

Ingredients

- 225g Watercress roughly chopped
- 2 cloves garlic roughly chopped
- 1Red Onion diced
- 2 tbsp olive oil
- 1-2 tbsp bouillon vegetable stock
- 300 - 400ml hot water (to mix stock in)
- Soy milk / cream / silken tofu / lemon optional if needed

Method

1. Mix the stock in the hot water. Sauté onions, garlic and oil on a med-high heat for about 5 minutes add stock (don't use all the stock, keep some behind and add at the end if needed) add watercress, put the lid on and simmer for 20 minutes.

2. If you find the watercress flavour too strong and the soup too runny, you could add some milk, cream or silken tofu at the end once tasted and seasoned to soften the taste and thicken the soup. I just added lemon juice to mine and poured some cream over the soup when served

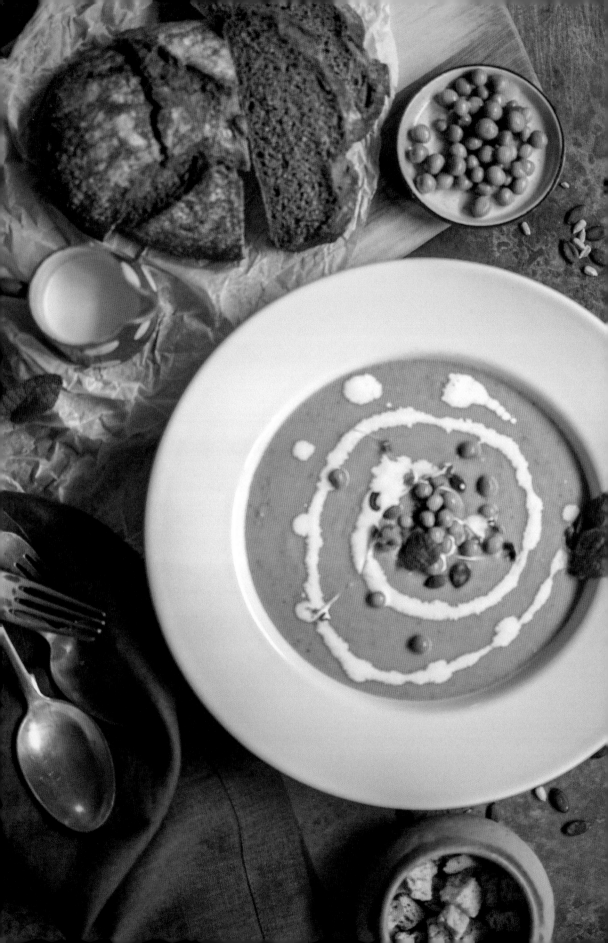

Pea & Mint Soup

Serves 4

Ingredients

- 1 large potato peeled and diced
- 5-6 sprigs of fresh mint / 2 tsp mint sauce
- 750g frozen peas (defrosted for best result)
- 2tbsp olive oil
- 1 large onion diced
- 3 gloves garlic roughly chopped
- 1-2 tbsp bouillon stock
- 500 ml hot water (Mix stock in) more water if needed after blending
- Salt and pepper to taste
- Cream to drizzle optional
- Asparagus to garnish/ serve with soup optional

Method

1. Mix stock into water and set aside. Place the onions, garlic, oil and half the mint in a pan on a med to high heat and sauté for 2-3 minutes. Now add the stock and potato and turn down to a med heat for 20 min.

2. Check if the potatoes are nearly ready and then add the peas and the rest of the mint and simmer for a further 5 minutes.

3. Don't cook for longer as you will lose the vibrant green colour of the peas. Using a hand blender or food processor, blend the soup to desired texture, add more water if it's too thick.

4. Season and serve with lemon or cream and asparagus.

Tip :

Defrost your peas beforehand so that they don't need longer than 5 min to cook at the end and keep their lovely vibrant colour.

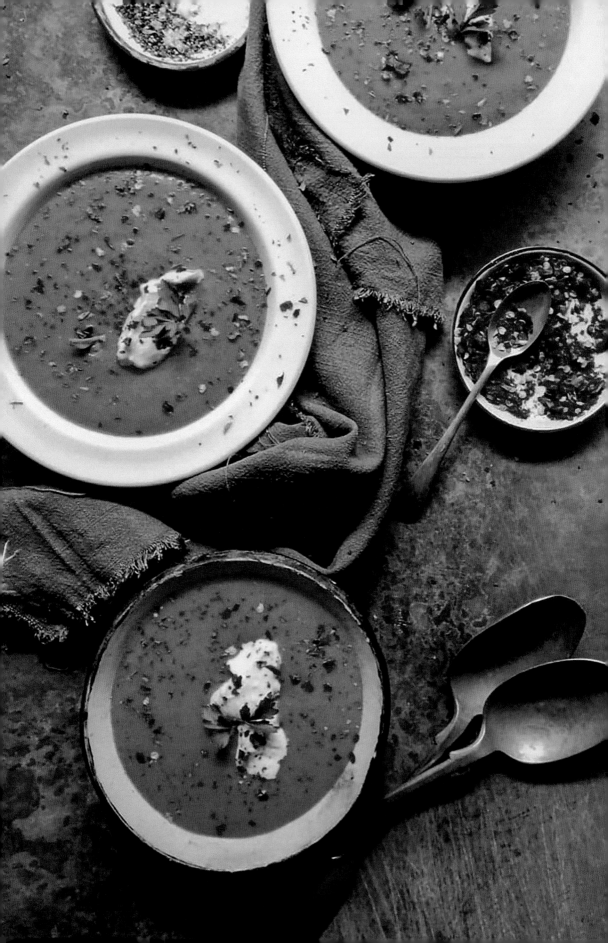

Roasted Red Peppers, Tomato & Chilli Soup

Serves 4-6

Perfect for winter especially English winters, hence why I add chillies to my soups! This is a lovely combination I came up with at work one day and I find it's really good for when I feel under the weather. Chillies, for me, seem to fight off any winter blues or sore throat. I simply can't have a winter without chillies! I added silken tofu to this for thickness and protein.

Ingredients

- 6 Large / 8 Med Tomatoes quartered
- 1 Red Onion roughly chopped
- 2 Tbsp Olive Oil
- 2 Garlic cloves roughly chopped
- Salt & Pepper to taste
- 1 Tsp Chilli Flakes (Optional)
- 480g Jar Char grilled Red Peppers drained and roughly chopped
- (349g) 1 box Silken Tofu (Blended Smooth)
- 350 ml warm water to make stock
- 1 Tbsp Bouillon Vegetable stock

Method

1. Mix the Bouillon with the warm water and stir well. Sauté onions, garlic, chilli flakes, tomatoes and oil in a large pot on med to high heat for 5 minutes. Stir occasionally then add in the red peppers and stir for a minute.

2. Pour in the stock; put the lid on, turn to medium heat and leave for another 5 minutes. Using a hand blender or a blender put the tofu in a bowl, blend till silky smooth.

3. Remove the pot from the heat, add the tofu into the soup and blend everything together till smooth. Add salt and pepper to taste.

Printed in Great Britain
by Amazon